Personal Assistance

Personal Assistance

THE FUTURE OF HOME CARE

Robert Morris, Francis G. Caro & John E. Hansan

The Johns Hopkins University Press ✸ *Baltimore & London*

© 1998 The Johns Hopkins University Press
All rights reserved. Published 1998
Printed in the United States of America on acid-free paper

9 8 7 6 5 4 3 2 1

The Johns Hopkins University Press
2715 North Charles Street
Baltimore, Maryland 21218-4363
The Johns Hopkins Press Ltd., London
www.press.jhu.edu

Library of Congress Cataloging-in-Publication Data will be found
at the end of this book.
A catalog record for this book is available from the British Library.

ISBN 0-8018-5902-6
ISBN 0-8018-5903-4 (pbk.)

Contents

Foreword

$\mathcal{A}$s the population of the United States continues, inexorably, to age and as the effects of modern medical care contribute to increasing longevity and the postponement of disability, there is a growing mismatch between the needs of the frailest and most dependent elderly individuals and the services available to them. What the disabled elderly (as well as the disabled nonelderly) most need is humane, responsive personal care provided in the communities where they live and prefer overwhelmingly to remain. What they can get, instead—if they get anything at all—is watered-down health care. While public health insurance programs contort themselves in the effort to adjust their presumably medical benefits to meet the nonmedical needs of their clients, hundreds of thousands, if not millions, of Americans go each day without the minimal help they need to perform what are quite literally the basic activities of daily living.

It's not as though these unmet needs are such a mystery. Indeed, for more than a decade, service providers and policymakers alike have recognized precisely where the most serious gaps in the system could be found. But in an era of profound political dissensus about social policy, both programmatic and policy development have been stalemated by a kind of chicken-and-egg standoff: without an assured funding base, service providers have been unwilling to reconfigure their activities to meet the needs of their clients or potential clients more directly; without satisfactory, high-quality, easily replicable models in place, policymakers have been unwilling to expand the funding base.

It's time to break that stalemate. Robert Morris, Francis Caro, and John Hansan have taken the critical first step by providing the most systematic and comprehensive effort yet undertaken to define exactly what it is that the frail and disabled most desperately need, and by describing how it could be gotten to them. By making personal assistance the focus of their analysis, Morris, Caro, and Hansan are able to explore not only what needs to be done, but how to do it.

One need not agree with everything in this book—I certainly don't—to be convinced that its authors have performed a vital service in setting the agenda for moving personal care forward. They deserve special praise for their emphasis on the need to design and build an appropriate infrastructure within which responsive, high-quality, efficient services could be provided. Such institutional development may make less exciting reading than characterizing needs or engaging in grand policy theory, but it is indeed the critical missing link in the development of a functioning and effective system of personal care for those who need it. Almost fifty years have passed since the Commission on Chronic Illness, to which the authors point so approvingly, but if we've learned anything in that time about efforts to develop long-term care services or policy, it is that institutional infrastructure matters at least as much as service definition or financing policy. No matter how sound the policy or sophisticated the caregivers, the right kinds of institutions will provide good services; the wrong institutions won't.

Whether, as a society, we will have the will and the wherewithal to build better institutions as part of the process of better addressing the needs of a burgeoning number of frail and disabled persons is an open and discomfiting question. But we will no longer have the excuse that we don't know what to do or don't know how to begin the process of moving forward. Morris, Caro, and Hansan have removed that excuse. For that, we all owe them our thanks.

Bruce C. Vladeck
Professor of Health Policy
The Mt. Sinai Medical Center
New York, New York

Preface

$\mathcal{W}$ITH THIS BOOK, we undertake the challenge of describing how formal personal assistance services can be organized, financed, and delivered efficiently and effectively to functionally disabled persons, thereby augmenting and extending the care provided by family and friends. The future of formal personal assistance arrangements will depend not only on government support but also on out-of-pocket payments by individuals and families and increasingly by cash benefits from affordable private insurance policies that emphasize home care over institutional care. We describe in detail in subsequent chapters the unique "window of opportunity" we have for addressing some of the barriers and shortcomings that have prevented personal assistance from developing into a full partner in the long-term-care continuum.

In the first three chapters, we establish the context for our analysis. In chapter 1, we trace the evolution of home and community care in the United States from its European origins. We pay particular attention to the federal long-term care initiatives in recent decades that focused first on institutional care and then expanded to include personal assistance in noninstitutional settings.

In chapter 2, we call attention to the scope and complexity of personal assistance needs by reporting on the prevalence of long-term disabling conditions and showing the diversity of their origins among people of all ages. The varied origins of personal assistance needs are significant because service interventions historically have been affected greatly by the age and diagnosis of those requiring initial medical care with personal assistance. Interventions that are focused on personal assistance needs apart from their origins are relatively recent and incomplete.

In chapter 3, we examine the family as the major provider of personal assistance. We consider both the strengths and limitations of families as sources of assistance. Recognition of the situations in which families cannot be expected to provide care leads to consideration of the ways in which families can call upon formal services to complement the assistance they themselves provide.

Chapter 4 is devoted to workforce issues. Because personal assistance is inherently labor intensive, the workers who assist the disabled with their daily living needs are at the heart of formal service systems. Historically, entry-level workers with limited training, modest supervision, and low wages have been deployed as personal assistance workers. Complaints about performance have often focused on the limitations of these workers. Efforts to improve formal services require that the workforce be upgraded. But, at the same time, efforts to contain personal assistance costs challenge the need to improve compensation for workers.

Much of our attention is on strategies to extend the effectiveness of formal services at modest cost. In chapter 5, we examine direct cash payments as an alternative to formal services in programs financed by third parties. Strategies that give consumers greater control in the use of resources are intriguing because consumers may be able to make more cost-effective use of resources. Moreover, current initiatives to test the potential of consumer-directed strategies should also instruct us about the circumstances in which conventionally managed services are more appropriate.

In chapter 6, we examine assistive devices as complements to human assistance. Our emphasis is on low-cost devices that permit those with self-care limitations to manage daily living needs more independently and more effectively. Particularly in the case of older people whose self-care limitations have developed gradually, we suspect that there is great potential for expansion in the use of devices to assist with bathing, dressing, meal preparation, and the like.

In chapter 7, we consider the potential for extending the effectiveness of assistance and controlling costs through more extensive use of volunteers. Although many formal services in the United States began as volunteer efforts, professionals now tend to be skeptical about volunteers as resources. Yet, volunteering continues to be widespread, and the potential for increasing volunteering, especially among retirees, is substantial. In light of the pressures to improve services without increasing costs and the tradition of volunteering in this country, we examine the potential for more extensive contributions by volunteers.

In chapter 8, we examine the relationship between personal assistance and health care. Because the need for assistance often originates with illness or injury, health care funds, notably Medicare and Medicaid, are often drawn on to finance personal assistance. Advocates for personal assistance often look to health care insurers as the potential source of more extensive financing of personal assistance. For these reasons, an understanding of the relationship between health care and personal assistance is essential to understanding both the organization of those services and their financing.

For many consumers, assisted living (chap. 9) has emerged as an important strategy and a welcome compromise between independent living and institutional care. Assisted living promises to provide safe, comfortable housing, permits efficient delivery of care and yet allows residents to retain substantial privacy and autonomy. The growth of assisted living also challenges home care providers to give assistance that is as comprehensive at a competitive price.

Financing (chap. 10) is central to any discussion of the future of personal assistance. We review current public and private sources of financing, the limitations of current financing, various proposals for improved financing, and their prospects. We emphasize the need for expanded attention on the part of growing numbers of middle-class consumers to financing through private insurance and out-of-pocket payments.

In chapter 11, we examine the roles of professionals in personal assistance. Focusing particularly on case managers, we contrast the established role case managers play in publicly financed programs with the more expansive role they can play in the growing private market.

In our conclusions, we offer our vision of the future of personal assistance in this country.

A glossary defines some of the terms and funding sources commonly used in connection with personal assistance and home care.

Acknowledgments

$\mathcal{T}$HIS BOOK COMBINES the integration of several years' experience and three years of writing in time stolen from responsibilities in a changing era for the academy. We are grateful for the help, sharing, and criticisms received over these years from colleagues too numerous to mention at Brandeis University, the University of Massachusetts–Boston, and others. But we also want to acknowledge the opportunities that these institutions gave us to think and test and experiment.

We want to acknowledge especially the help we received over the past three years from Wendy Harris, medical editor at the Johns Hopkins University Press. She was by turns encouraging, critical, and generous in sharing ideas. Rosalie Cordwell, R.N., and many others at the Visiting Nurse Association of Boston provided us with numerous examples of what can be done to secure a normal life in a home of one's own for chronically ill, aged, or disabled people.

We wish to thank Josephine Sturgis for clerical assistance and Terri Salmons for research assistance. We are also grateful to Charlotte Fritz and Alison Gottleib for their critical reading of portions of the manuscript. In addition, we are appreciative of the financial support from the Gerontology Institute, University of Massachusetts–Boston, and from Capitol Advantage, McLean, Virginia.

Finally, our wives—Sara, Carol, and Ethel—not only were long-suffering but also actively helped in many ways, from encouragement to research to technical help to accepting our time sequestered at the computer.

Personal Assistance

Introduction

$\mathcal{F}$AMILIES ARE and will continue to be the major providers of personal assistance for an aged parent or other family member with physical or mental limitations. But there are a growing number of instances in which a functionally disabled person does not have a spouse or family member available to help over an extended length of time. What happens? Where can they go for help? This book examines the issues involved when a noninstitutionalized youth or adult requires the help of someone other than a family member or friend in managing the everyday activities of living (Vladeck 1980).

The extent of the need for personal assistance with of daily life is a measure of a person's ability to live independently. When it is necessary to go outside oneself or one's family to obtain assistance in managing everyday activities—dressing, bathing, cooking, eating, shopping, chores, transportation, and the like—there are essentially only three options: buy what is needed, obtain it from a public agency or charity, or go without. This book focuses on how formal personal assistance services provided in an individual's home, purchased through direct employment or supplied by an organization of some kind, can complement the care provided by family members and friends.

The array of medical and personal care services that are required by chronically ill or disabled persons over a significant length of time are referred to as the long-term-care (LTC) continuum. In the continuum, home care stands opposite from institutional care, commonly represented by nursing homes. Against measures such as personal satisfaction or costs, home care is far preferable to institutional care, except in the most severe cases of functional disability or where there is a need for specialized equipment or security. Evidence of this preference can be seen in the increased popularity of assisted living arrangements that allow elderly persons and others who are at risk to live in a home environment while depending on the management to provide meals, cleaning, transportation, security, and other services.

Home care, sometimes called community-based care, consists of a range of

supportive and personal assistance services that persons with functional disabilities receive in their homes from outside sources. Generally speaking, home-
and community-based long-term care can be classified as either personal assistance services or community services. Examples of personal assistance include
bathing, meal preparation, housework, and transportation. Examples of community services include meals delivered to the home, congregate meals, senior
centers, adult day care, and respite care.

Our focus is directed primarily at the options available for locating, financing, organizing, and supervising personal care activities provided by someone
other than a close family member, relative, or friend. This is a significant area of
inquiry for several reasons: (1) the number of functionally disabled persons is
growing very rapidly; (2) the capacity of families to provide all the personal care
required by elderly parents and other physically or mentally disabled members
over a long period of time is being reduced by a number of significant social and
economic changes; and (3) the enormous cost of our traditional public (and
charitable) responses to this issue will be financially insupportable in the very
near future unless some changes are made in the way we organize and pay for
tax-supported long-term care.

With this book, we attempt to disentangle overlapping concepts and briefly
describe the most influential organizational structures, sources of funding, and
professional staff interests that shape the current provision of long-term personal care to chronically ill, feeble elderly, and other functionally disabled persons. We also describe and clarify the concepts that differentiate the service links
that form our present system of long-term care. We demonstrate how a succession of public policies and institutional vested interests have combined to create our current publicly financed and very expensive long-term-care system
built almost entirely on nursing home care. It is notable mainly for the fact that
it "institutionalized and medicalized" routine personal assistance and social supports at a very great cost to taxpayers. At the same time, the system leaves many
who have extensive self-care limitations and modest financial resources with
little or no affordable assistance.

Long-term-care services, especially those that are home- and community-
based, have recently come to the fore as public policy concerns because of a
distinct set of human needs, important demographic and social changes, and
increasing specialization in health care and social services. But long-term care
has always lacked a conceptual foundation that public policy analysts and public officials can draw on to shape its development adequately. Advocacy for
improvements in long-term-care financing and long-term-care services has relied on loosely formulated rationales and incremental reforms—strategies that

have not worked well in the competition for public resources with such sectors as health care for poor or elderly persons.

At the heart of a long-term-care system is an array of personal services for assisting functionally disabled persons with the activities of daily living they cannot manage alone. Conceptually, long-term care is distinct from health care, which treats acute or chronic medical needs of disabled persons. Long-term care is also distinct from convalescence and rehabilitation services, which seek restoration in functioning. We emphasize that long-term care is distinct from other intervention systems in order to assure that the domain is addressed.

The most widely used construct with which to identify functional limitation is that of an activities of daily living scale. There are variations in items to be included. Conventionally these are listed: getting in and out of bed, toileting, bathing, dressing, and eating. The degree of limitaion is determined by observation of family, an aide, or a clinician, or by self-report. The number of functions reported as limited are added up to give a rough measure of severity. This scale is supplemented by an instrumental activity scale covering limitations in performing such tasks as taking medications, preparing meals, doing light housework, using a telephone, and being able to get in and out of the house, which are important for life at home.

Long-term care should have a set of objectives that is independent of the setting in which it is provided. The primary aim of long-term care is to assure adequate solutions to problems of daily living for functionally disabled persons, frail elders, Alzheimer's disease patients—anyone who has physical or mental limitations that prevent independent living. Functionally disabled persons should have the opportunity to approximate living experiences that are consistent with age norms in their society. Another purpose of long-term-care services, for example, may be to provide relief to informal care providers. A humane society may set limits to the caregiving responsibilities expected of relatives. Personal assistance services, respite care, and adult day care are all examples of long-term-care services that are available to reduce the effort expected of those caregiving family members who exceed that limit.

The current model for long-term care assumes a seamless web of affordable health care and personal services, including hospital and physician treatments through skilled nursing care, rehabilitation, and personal assistance necessary to cope with lifelong disability. This model conceals as much as it reveals. A long-term-care cycle usually proceeds through three phases, but not mechanically: phase 1 is a short period (a few days or weeks) in which medical care is dominant and is usually provided in a hospital setting; phase 2, variously called subacute care, extended care, or convalescent care, is the period in which recovery requires *both* medical care and personal care and may last for several weeks or months; phase 3 is the phase in which personal assistance in some form is dominant because of long-term physical dependency due to severe physical or mental disability or chronic illness.

The popular conception of long-term care is distorted because the costs of acute medical care services are largely insured by employers and the government. Seldom do third-party payers help with the costs of home care or personal assistance, and then under strict limitations. Personal assistance is the weakest link in the long-term-care continuum, with the least public support and the smallest share of the long-term-care dollar.

Personal assistance remains underdeveloped because of limited public financing, limited consumer purchasing power, weaknesses in the organization of formal assistance services, and lack of consumer confidence in those services. Nevertheless, notwithstanding the current reality, personal assistance is the component of long-term care that presents the greatest potential for helping a large proportion of the disabled and very frail population lead as normal a life as possible. The question is: how can a social support service so common to family life become better organized and more available to help meet the anticipated growth in the number of persons with disabling conditions?

CHAPTER 1 ❈ *Early and Recent Evolution of Home and Community Care*

CARE OF VERY SICK, disabled, or frail aged persons has concerned all societies to some degree from the beginning of recorded history. Only a few documents directly, and some literature indirectly, hint at how early Western societies cared for their handicapped and dependent members from the biblical period until the enactment of the poor laws in England and Western Europe in the fourteenth century. It is clear from these sources that the family took care of its own. It was easier for the wealthy minority in Greece and Rome, with their slave or client followers, to do all that could be done—helped, perhaps, by the fact that the average life expectancy was short, 30–40 years for most, although a few people lived to old age. Without evidence, we can only assume that the poor took care of each other as best they could.

Jewish and Christian biblical teaching enjoined families, friends, and neighbors to look after one another (Morris 1986). The major public responsibility was to assure that all the poor had a minimum amount of grain and oil for food. Philanthropy as then understood was usually for one's peers as a kind of gift that was to be reciprocated. It was not for the poor. If the wealthy gave to the poor, it was for their basic sustenance. During the medieval period, the teachings of the Roman Catholic Church encouraged the faithful to "care for the needy" and "do unto others what you would have them do unto you." Early church views about charity encouraged the development of hostels and hospices, usually for travelers but also to receive the poor and beggars, many of whom were handicapped. Over the centuries secular foundations also evolved, encouraged by church doctrines about one's responsibility to help the poor, the sick, and the orphaned. Some were formed by craft guilds to provide a little security for families of their deceased members, usually in the form of money or goods in kind, always as religiously sanctioned charity.

Societies are known to have accommodated the needs of their physically and mentally dependent members in various ways. The nature of the help provided individuals without the protection of family or wealth took different forms, depending largely on the values and resources of the community. For example, when the Black Death reduced the population of England almost 25 percent in 1348–49, there followed a period of social and economic unrest when large numbers of people left their traditional homes and farms in search of higher wages and better opportunities.

The conditions of this period in English history contributed to a significant increase in the number of vagabonds and roving gangs engaged in unlawful activities. It became difficult for citizens to distinguish between an able-bodied stranger genuinely in need of help and one intent on looting or doing violence. To help the populace cope with these conditions, the first English law of settlement was enacted in 1388. Under the terms of this law, able-bodied beggars were subject to punishment, but those *unable to work* (the aged, feeble-minded, blind, disabled, etc.) were permitted to beg, though only at their current place of residence or the place where they were born.

Subsequent English poor laws further reinforced this distinction between those unable to work as the "worthy" poor and the able-bodied as "unworthy" poor. This is important for two reasons: the systems of caring for dependent persons that evolved in the United States were heavily influenced by the values and practices incorporated in the English poor laws; and orphans, aged widows, the blind, and physically disabled persons needing financial support continued to be viewed as "worthy poor" entitled to some level of public assistance.

Poor Laws and Poorhouses

Throughout history, the majority of aged and disabled persons needing care or personal assistance received it from family members, provided according to the values and mores of their time and social condition. Wealthy people, with or without family support, have usually been able to purchase the medical care and personal assistance services they required, if it was available. It is only when long-term care or personal assistance services for the aged and disabled require taxpayer support that they become a matter of public discussion and policy making. Such was the case in England during the late 1500s, when industrialization, worker dislocation, and famine combined to create a high degree of involuntary unemployment. The rise in the number of vagrants and beggars swamped the ability of monasteries and other religious groups to respond to the pleas for help.

To cope with the "begging nuisance," more and more communities created secular authorities to empower an "overseer of the poor" whose job it was to administer the distribution of relief to the needy. The epitome of this trend toward relying on public authority was reached with enactment of the first Elizabethan Poor Law (1597–1601), the first set of completely secular guidelines for how local communities were to treat economically dependent people. With later revisions Poor Laws remained in effect for nearly two hundred and fifty years and, in many respects, continue to influence public values about how and in what fashion the poor and other dependent persons should be treated. The two most significant and enduring aspects of the Elizabethan Poor Law are (1) that it placed on local governments the legal obligation to raise taxes in order to care for the poor, if and when local voluntary charity was insufficient; and (2) that it identified three categories of dependents—the vagrant, the involuntary unemployed, and the helpless. The articulation of these categories allowed public officials to distinguish between the worthy and unworthy poor and how to deal with each population.

The major institution that emerged was the poorhouse, where anyone who became economically or physically dependent could be housed. It dumped together the poor, debtors, widows, and orphans—all who lacked a family or money to care for themselves. While benevolent in intention, poorhouses were quickly undermined when local tax funds were diverted for other purposes. Despite numerous reform efforts, the poorhouses and the poor laws became synonymous with cruelty, neglect, and abuse.

The Era of Scientism and Political Reform

From its founding, the United States patterned care and treatment of the aged and disabled on the English tradition, with heavy reliance on the poorhouse. The growing prosperity and increased urbanization that followed the Civil War led to pressures for public institution reforms and an increase in private charities to help the poor. Almost all attention was given to relieving gross economic destitution. Private philanthropies increased and gradually became professional. A persistent and troublesome debate was carried on over "indoor versus outdoor relief"—whether to provide help only to dependent residents, making them live in an institution of some kind, or to give a small amount of cash to those who could continue to live at home.

Spurred by the influence of scientism and the power of rationality, reformers, physicians, and, later, public health workers pushed for new approaches and reforms appeared in connection with public health and prevention of communicable diseases. Citizen movements in public and mental health fostered the construction of special state-financed and -administered hospitals for the so-called incurable and asylums for the mentally ill. Confidence grew that society could build "ideal" communities for the mentally ill as an alternative to the harsh realities of the Industrial Revolution—that scientific methods would conquer the most disturbing mental ills (Rothman 1956). Such communicable diseases as tuberculosis, then a major killer, could be managed by public health prevention measures that ranged from isolation in sanatoria during treatment, to quarantine measures at home, to major housing efforts designed to abolish the unhealthy living conditions of the poor, primarily new immigrants.

Public health became a major new profession dealing with a healthy environment—clean water, sewage disposal, and the like. Public health nurses visited poor families (mainly but not exclusively) to teach them the principles of healthy living and personal care. While such efforts were designed to reduce death rates among women in childbirth and the premature death of newborn infants, the educational reach was much broader. A movement was initiated to increase public understanding about mental illness as a treatable disease. Families continued to take care of their sick and disabled members, but those most threatening to social health could be removed to institutions and humanely treated with modern methods (Rothman 1956).

Such public programs were paralleled by nonprofit, charitable initiatives; rest homes, convalescent homes, and homes for the aged were developed by religious and ethnic groups and by philanthropic agencies urged on by a growing Victorian sensibility that the newly wealthy of the industrial era had a private responsibility for the disadvantaged of society. Family and children's service agencies sprang up. Staff of these organizations became witness to many health and social needs, some of which they tried to manage, mostly problems of poverty and ignorance. Moreover their evidence about social and health needs led others to support public efforts to administer or finance health care institutions and hospitals and to wipe out slums. (Chambers 1963; Lubov 1962).

By midcentury, physicians began to visit patients at home more often. Public health nurses visited families to give instruction or to give nursing care at home, at least for acute illness. Organized home care was incorporated in a pioneer program at University Hospital, Boston University, with student interns visiting the poor at home to provide medical care as part of their education. This trend declined later on as medical therapies became more complex and physicians chose hospitals as the preferred site for treatment. But the number of surviving patients with long-term chronic illness increased to the point that the beds they occupied were needed for patients who could recover with new therapies. To make room, chronic patients were discharged to various alternative settings—families, chronic specialty hospitals and sanatoria, private ethnic or religious congregate homes, mutual aid societies, and boarding homes. In some cases (e.g., Philadelphia), a chronic facility was built adjoining an acute care hospital, which administered it. The opportunity to develop a unified, comprehensive hospital acute plus long-term care system passed; the private homes of several kinds became the foundation for what were later called "nursing homes," with a distinct medical and nursing orientation.

The Children's Bureau was established as part of the U.S. Department of Labor in 1912, the first federal agency directly concerned with individual civilians' welfare. Its mission was at first limited to reports on the conditions of children that warranted public attention. It become a major influence in developing health care and social services under public auspices, including services for crippled children.

The family remained the basic source of care for the handicapped and aged. The wealthy could afford comfortable sanatoria. The poor and those without family had last resort access to rigorous means-tested poorhouses or to some private charity homes. Since average life expectancy was about 40 there was not yet much recognition that disability and old age would become major problems for society as well as for communities and for families. In the meantime, earlier patterns—institutions for the "deserving poor" and "poorhouses" for the rest— persisted, ameliorated somewhat by private efforts to educate poor families in self care or to remove those seen as threatening to health or peace of mind to specialized medical public institutions or asylums.

The Progressive Era, the period between 1900 and the end of World War I, is notable as the "seed time for reform." It was a period during which ideas and programs for better ways to provide for the disadvantaged, especially the handicapped, were first conceived. The early concern for developing new and more humane programs was nurtured by confidence in the future of science and technology, in improved health as well as in manufacture, and in the authority of government—federal, state, and local—to act in the interest of citizens' well-being when the private sector could not or would not. Government was seen as the necessary corrective to the consequences of the demographic, industrial, and urbanizing trends of the twentieth century.

Until 1935, the benefits of these new developments were limited to the residents of only a few states. Among the new developments were state-financed programs to assure a minimum income for certain groups, such as retirement benefits for elderly workers, mother's pensions, workmen's compensation, and the like. A number of these state programs served as the models for enactment of the Social Security Act in 1935. For example, the Social Security Act created a set of contributory social insurance programs intended to protect working individuals and their families who found themselves unable to work through no fault of their own: unemployment insurance, old age and survivors insurance, and later, insurance for the permanently disabled. In the succeeding thirty years a buoyant and growing economy acted as the foundation for adding a wider range of social supports.

1945–1965

By 1946, building on experiences gleaned from a few pioneer experiments like that at Montefiore Hospital in New York City (see below), a Joint Committee on Chronic Disease began its work and reported in 1956 as the Commission on Chronic Illness. It developed a systematic argument in favor of the pivotal role that various supportive services could play, along with the private physician, in the care of the chronically ill. Homemakers and personal care staff were seen as crucial partners along with nurses, doctors, and other health professionals. Hospitals and nursing homes were no longer seen as the sole or primary resource for the chronically sick, although linkage between them was also necessary for short-term acute-care episodes. The report provided a conceptual foundation but did not offer an organizational blueprint. Neither did it then have available quantitative and evaluative data about nonhospital and social services, about changes in clinical conditions as patients moved form one site to another, or about details of costs now considered necessary to buttress demonstration experiences (Benjamin 1993; National Commission on Chronic Illness 1956).

The decline of the poorhouse was hastened by the Social Security Administration's denial of reimbursement to local public institutions for custodial care. Social Security payments, small as they were initially, encouraged retirement from the work force for those over 65. It promised a future of income security after the loss of private savings in the Depression, a future built on a restoration of the economy. Private rest homes and small boarding homes grew to replace sole reliance on a family home when population mobility and the increase of widowed and single elderly curtailed the utility of the family. Retired nurses often found new private careers during the Depression by opening their homes to a few boarders, some of whom needed supportive help beyond mere shelter.

After World War II there was an era of economic expansion, with increase in gross national product and in federal tax income produced by a vigorous economy. Congress had available new funds to finance new social programs in response to growing citizen demands (Hansan and Morris 1997).

Studies by Jarrett and Boas publicized the problems of the chronically sick and noted that home services of the time were limited to convalescent care and limited to children. At first chronic disease hospitals were seen as the alternative (Jarrett 1933a, b; Boas 1930). Others argued that home care was both less costly and a better place to treat such conditions (Bardwell 1930; Epstein 1930). Cost and adequacy of the home environment divided proponents of alternative policies.

Nursing homes developed rapidly after 1945 as new therapeutic methods increased the survival of the severely disabled whose needs exceeded the capacity of a boarding home. Shortage of hospital beds speeded the trend to free hospital beds for acute care, and the need for new institutions for chronic care surfaced. Social Security benefits, plus rising incomes of two-worker families, promised the financial means for an enterprise that could be both a community service and profitable. Profit-making homes grew, as did nonprofit home capacity, by modernizing homes for the aged.

This was also the time when the clinical and rehabilitation experiences in World War II and the speedy evolution of new drug and surgical procedures combined to increase the survival rate of the severely sick or disabled. Rehabilitation became an important medical specialty. And progress in the life sciences opened new approaches to treating or managing progressive neurological and developmental diseases.

In 1946 the Hill-Burton Act stimulated construction of hospitals in all parts of the country to treat the acutely ill who could be restored to full or partial health and returned more quickly to community life. The changes in technology increased the survival of those of all ages who could return to some non-hospital existence but would needed both recurrent medical attention and social supports. A dramatic example was the methods developed out of World War II to keep alive and treat victims spinal cord injuries. Young and old who once would have died in a year now survived with the disability for many years. Similarly, antibiotics conquered many pulmonary ills like pneumonia, which once caused death in middle and early old age. It had the effect, too, of increasing the survival rate of older persons, who, in time, would become more feeble and less able to manage without some support other than a doctor's visit.

In 1950, Old Age Assistance (OAA), part of the public welfare programs created with the Social Security Act of 1935, authorized matching payments by state and local welfare agencies for health and social services supplied by vendors. Limited OAA funds began to make it easier for poor recipients of OAA to continue living in their own homes rather than in a county home. It helped local welfare departments extend homemaker services to the aged for longer periods of time, going beyond the earlier public programs of short-term home-maker services for sick mothers following hospitalization or those with new-born infants.

The Social Security Administration did explore the innovative comprehensive home-care experiments pioneered as early as the 1930s by New York's Monte-fiore Hospital, which developed a program that included use of physician super-vision, nurses, aides, and homemakers. It concentrated on the chronic patients' long-term social and medical needs in an integrated program beyond the need to move them out of the hospital quickly. Service continued as long as the patient required help to remain at home, and staff had wide discretion in deciding what combination of services was needed (Benjamin 1993). This open-ended, patient-focused experiment seemed to budget-sensitive public officials to open the door to uncontrolled expansion of services beyond the mission or resources of Medi-care as then envisioned.

Visiting nurse associations and some local health departments had also devel-oped home-care services using nurses, nurses aides, and homemakers (house-keepers). At first these were seen as private charity responsibilities. Until the 1950s most of these services were for time-limited episodes following hospi-talization. Initially, most home-care services concentrated on family education for health care and on caring for children and convalescents. Many of these patients were recent immigrants, indigent, or poor, and there was little evidence of middle-class interest. The agencies had not yet entered the medical world, where rigorous cost management became the criterion and "businesslike" prac-tices dominated administration. Health insurance, especially through Blue Cross in several states, did try to cover home-care services but within very con-stricting rules: eligible patients had to be accepted directly on discharge from a hospital and need services for a limited period; hospital supervision was deemed necessary; intermittent services to the home were limited and usually included only medically related specialties under physician supervision. The number of visits was sharply limited. If a patient was ambulatory, it was argued that a med-ical center visit for attention was cheaper, ignoring the social support needs of those with chronic disability. The same restrictions were retained in Medicare. Chronic care continued to be closely tied to the medical facility and its per-spectives. Nevertheless, visiting nurse associations and public health depart-ments, where personal care and other social supports were deemed as important as medical treatment, were becoming visible supporters of home-care alterna-tives. Medicaid, Medicare, and private fee reimbursements replaced most of the charity-based forms of support (Benjamin 1993; Follman 1963; Jarrett 1933a, b).

The concentration on institutional care in public policy continued through the federal mortgage or loan guarantee program. Guarantees were authorized to proprietary institutions in 1954, and in 1956 and 1959 such loan insurance was authorized through the Federal Housing Authority ($1 billion at first).

The 1950s also saw a renewed effort to enact national health insurance that failed. The health insurance debates did, however, lead to an expansion of the Hill-Burton Hospital Construction Act to include nonprofit and public nursing homes "built in conjunction with a hospital." This language was sufficiently vague that the link between hospital and nursing home was left unclear. But the effect was to encourage a parallel system of care with a strong leaning toward a medical model of institutional care for the disabled. What began as a custodial institution for helpless individuals without family care became more and more a medically oriented institution for care following hospitalization.

With an assured source for referrals (hospitals) and more assured public and private financing, a new industry—the proprietary nursing home—grew rapidly and became the major nonfamily resource. The rudiments of a progressive care system were begun, stretching from hospital, to family or convalescent care of either short- or long-term duration, to nursing home for the long-term (custodial) care, if not to family.

The Great Society Era

The Kerr-Mills bill proposed to expand federal coverage for medical care to the "medically indigent"—those who had too much income to pass a means text but not enough to pay for medical care. It was a delaying action to efforts to enact a national health insurance plan. The bill was soon supplanted by enactment of both Medicaid and Medicare, which extended essential medical care to the elderly without means testing. The Kerr-Mills debate paved the way for including federal matching funds for ten home health care services, leaving the decision up to individual states (Coll 1995).

Medicare was federally controlled; Medicaid divided responsibility between federal and state governments. Each tried to deal with the combination of rising costs and dissatisfactions with nursing home care. The efforts concentrated initially on controls in nursing homes rather than alternative care modalities. For this time the choice was inevitable, given the rapid growth of an extensive nursing home system with large capital investments and ideological and practice links to medicine. Home care had a place in the national debate, but it was limited by Medicare's medical and posthospital responsibilities; Medicare became a large payer for home care, albeit of a medical variety (Weissert et al. 1988; Callender 1975; Lavor 1979).

Despite limited policy actions for home care, the debate leading to the enactment of Medicare and Medicaid did raise the level of national awareness about home care. This evolution was furthered by the fact that Medicare, as a way to control hospital costs, provided up to 120 days of nursing home care for patients whom hospitals could not or would not keep.

The debate leading to the enactment of Medicare introduced legislative committees to home care just when they were trying to reconcile conflicting public pressures to control escalating medical costs and to expand access to more medical care. Thus the formula was adopted to permit use of Medicare dollars for a few days of nursing home care in order "to give extended post hospital care" to patients who needed nursing attention but not necessarily in a hospital. The obvious resource for such limited care became the nursing home. It took several years to incorporate funding for comparable care at home, even for a short time (Risse et al. 1977; Benjamin 1993; Follman 1963).

In January 1975 a new social services block grant to the states was authorized by Title XX of the Social Security Act, authorizing expenditures up to $2.5 billion in federal funds so that welfare clients and other low-income persons could achieve five national goals, one of which was: "prevention and reduction of inappropriate institutionalization by providing community care services" (Hansan 1980). Subsequently, some of these funds were used to provide home and community services to help the chronically ill and disabled remain in their own homes.

Medicare continued to increase its coverage for medically linked home care. Medicaid, with its joint state and federal control, was as much a welfare program as a medical one. Title XX funds were administered by a social welfare, not a medical, agency, and Medicaid funds were not confined to "medically necessary" services. But throughout 1970–90 developments were driven by pressure to deal with rising medical and health costs. Even with marginal improvements in financing, home care remained a small ticket item overshadowed by the escalating costs of hospital, medical, and nursing home care—so much so that the medical perspective dominated actions and entitlement. Nursing homes continued to be seen as a complicated way, at best, to combat rising costs of hospital care.

Evidence about home care as a medically acceptable and cost effective alternative was not yet available. What became clear was that home care, even in a minor role, was now a part of the national debate even though Medicare criteria limited the use of public dollars to intermittent medical and nursing procedures for short periods after a hospital discharge (Green et al. 1993; Hughes 1985).

While Medicare continued to be a major payer for limited home care, a broader definition was being promoted during 1965–75 by the Office on Aging, by the many but weak and divided social service agencies, and by public health leaders. As minor changes were made in both Medicare and Medicaid laws, some states began to experiment with more flexible criteria for social home care. Since states could control most publicly supported nursing home admissions, some supported social home-care services, when deemed necessary, to delay or deter nursing home admissions on the grounds that home care was more economical for state budgets.

The discussion was hampered by conflicting evidence from poorly designed research, which could not replicate strong evidence that various form of home care could control health care costs, even if patients were happier at home. The most thorough analyses found that home care was only sometimes less costly and for more complex conditions was actually costlier (Weissert 1985). While home care grew its financing remained modest (Callender 1975; Lavor 1979).

Several other remedies for rising medical costs were initiated. Differential reimbursements based on level of care required was introduced for nursing homes but not for home care. Care was divided between skilled care, intermediate care, and other state formulations. Each level required different records and secured different payments—the higher the reported quality of care, the costlier the services, thus the higher the reimbursement. With patient conditions changing frequently, limited record-keeping, inadequate staffing, lack of on-site physician supervision, costs continued to escalate without effective controls either by regulation or by professional discipline.

As dissatisfactions persisted, other ideas were tried. In 1971 Professional Service Review Organizations were authorized in an attempt to control the use of costly medical procedures. Dissatisfactions still persisted. In 1974 the Department of Health, Education, and Welfare awarded contracts to compare outcomes of medical day care with homemaker programs. The results were difficult to interpret and required further research (Benjamin 1993).

In the 1970s concern about rising medical costs was joined with equal concern about rising nursing home costs and the unsatisfactory quality of services. The Levinson Policy Institute, Brandeis University, was established in 1971 and for ten years conducted analyses, demonstrations, and evaluations that concentrated on the social or functional approach to home care and its relation to health care (Morris 1971; Sager 1976).

The institute argued through legislative hearings and demonstrations that care at home was both more attractive and less (or at least not more) costly than the nursing home option. One approach, the personal care organization

(PCO), emphasized personal assistance services through a single organization that would take comprehensive responsibility for services. The PCO was an entity with which Medicaid could contract to provide personal assistance economically.

A report in 1973 (Caro 1973) laid out the main themes, of the development of home and community-based long-term care for two decades, but they remain unresolved in the 1990s:

❋ a feasible rationale for home care;

❋ personal assistance for all age groups;

❋ payment based on capitation, negotiated to reflect variations in functional disability;

❋ capitation based on standardized measures of functional disability;

❋ relationships with health and medical agencies;

❋ use of nonprofessional home helpers, their recruitment and retention;

❋ role of a case manager;

❋ potential for combining personal care organizations and health maintenance organizations;

❋ application to disability groups of all ages, including adult disabled, mentally ill, and retarded persons

The first demonstration was for a personal care organization undertaken with the Massachusetts Department of Welfare. It called for home care for elderly patients with disability, financed by state funds, with sliding scale fees, and the expectation that services would be intermittent but lengthy (U.S. Senate Special Committee on Aging 1971).

Demonstrations of a PCO were later launched through the lieutenant governor's office of Wisconsin, relying on the state and county welfare system to fund, administer, and evaluate alternative local public models. At the conclusion the recommendations were continued in modified form by the City of Milwaukee. In time and with other local studies, the PCO became the foundation for the later Wisconsin Community Options Program. This program provided state-appropriated funds to counties and allowed them to decide how to give their potential nursing home population a real choice in whether to remain at home or enter an institution. It is administered by each county with general monitoring of the distribution of specially appropriated funds. After frequent legislative reviews it has been found that the home-care option is slightly less costly than a nursing home choice; but, as the eligible population grows in size, the aggregate costs will increase. Unit costs prove less expensive (Spann 1987).

Similar demonstrations with different populations and different structures were initiated by others. The most widely quoted evaluations are those of Weissert (1985, 1988a, b, c), who found no conclusive evidence that substitution of home care for nursing home admission took place among those imminently at risk of entering a nursing home. Yet it has not been possible to find clear evidence that early home care will divert patients from entering a nursing home later. Cost savings have generally been mixed. Costs at home for *very* complex conditions can be at least as high as in a nursing home. Much home care economy results from fewer costly services that individuals may not need at home although they are provided for everyone in nursing homes, either to be competitive in attracting patients or to meet regulatory standards.

By 1977 a report of the Congressional Budget Office (CBO) slowed momentum. It concluded that a disproportionate share of public funding for the aged and adult disabled population was going to nursing homes, but it also cautioned that home care could become more costly than nursing home care (CBO 1977). The aging population, increased use of nursing homes, and rapid rise in use of home *medical* care led the General Accounting Office and others to note anxiety about "uncontrolled spending" (Derthick 1975, 1990; GAO 1992). Furthermore, proprietary agencies had entered the home-care provider market and quickly became major players in what had been a nonprofit cottage industry. Abuses in home-care services reported in congressional hearings made it clear that home care had "lost its innocence." The service was no longer a protected, well-intended philanthropy, but a boisterous health field in one of the nation's major "industries" (Benjamin 1993).

In 1980 the Levinson Policy Institute proposed a social maintenance organization (SMO) to complement the personal care organization model. The SMO is a model with Medicare reimbursements, under research contracts, for social support services planned and directed by physicians in health maintenance organizations (HMOs) as part of their treatment plan for a patient. The reimbursements were limited to total costs no higher than the average area expenditure or, at one stage, no more than 95 percent of the average. Ultimately, eight demonstrations were funded (Leutz 1994). Variations of this approach were developed independently by PACE (On Lok) and incorporated in legislation covering eighteen sites.

STATE OF THE ART IN THE 1990S

The National Channeling Demonstration project of 1979–85 is an example of a national effort to use research to find acceptable solutions to the contradictions. It established evidence that managing the flow from one site to another as a patient's condition changed could make some difference in what services were finally used, but the underlying difficulties were not resolved, only widely reported (Callahan 1996). It found that, as designed, no model was much used by those not already in imminent risk of going to a nursing institution. Costs were either increased or, in the aggregate, not reduced and the benefits, while measurable, were not considered significant (Weissert). Still, home care had assumed a firm if minor place in federal programs. Use of social services at home increased. Efforts at the margin were sufficiently valued by many to keep it going, but costs rose nevertheless and concern about erosion of family responsibility persisted.

Channeling, despite its failure to satisfy the need to control costs, contributed to the expansion of a constituency interested in home care—professionals, advocates, and families who became convinced of the merits of a solid home-care program. It contributed to the expansion of the federal waiver program, which shifted responsibility to new hands at the state level. While the consequences of channeling are still being debated, it has added to the growing variety of efforts to move on the home-care path.

By 1982, the idea of hospice was recognized in regulations governing Medicare reimbursement. Although an ancient service, hospice in its modern form began as a specialized institution for terminally ill patient whose needs could be defined as managing pain in the last days of life. Very soon, hospice services were brought to the patient at home, when the family was prepared to share in the pain of terminal care for the dying, a function that hospitals had long ago abandoned whenever they could. In 1982 legislation was enacted that provided strict guidelines and generous financing for the complex of terminal care services, some of which involved participation by relatives. By 1985 an estimated 150,000 patients were treated with hospice services in a year. By 1994, Medicare or Medicaid covered 300,000 patients at a public cost on average of $80 a day (Vladeck 1995; Shapiro 1994). Hospice enlarged interest in social home care.

By 1989 home health care had became Medicare's fastest growing (although still minor) program, costing $2 billion. Medicaid expenditures for more diverse social-medical home care quadrupled at the same time that public concern was growing that hospitals, in order to curtail costs, were discharging elderly prematurely and predominantly to nursing homes or to profit-making home-care corporations, which by 1991 served a third of Medicare-certified home-care agencies (Estes and Binney 1988).

By the 1990s both Medicare and Medicaid had become major sources of funds for home health and personal assistance, although Medicare still limited its support to cases of medical necessity for the time required to complete a course of treatment. Still, personal assistance and other social supports were increasingly funded for short periods of time. But when overall costs rose rapidly, the Medicare home-care program came under attack, and spending reductions were proposed. In Medicaid the funding remained linked to welfare eligibility and the risk of needing nursing home care.

Thus, support for personal assistance continued to grow, but within narrow ranges. The place of personal assistance in the development of a more comprehensive and effective long-term-care system designed to help people with disabilities live at home remains problematic. The long-term-care continuum is still largely incomplete.

The Robert Wood Johnson Foundation launched a demonstration project in public-private collaboration. Clients who purchased long-term-care insurance early enough (especially when the policies covered personal assistance as well as nursing home care) could protect their assets up to the amount of protection purchased in case the insured later was forced to apply for Medicaid (welfare eligibility). Four states passed authorizing legislation and interest in further expansion of private, affordable, long-term-care policies has increased.

These developments in a huge system divided among separately mandated programs were pushed to constant change by a combination of new technology, more demands for help, public resistance to high costs, and a growing array of stratagems even as the population aged and the numbers if not the proportion of the disabled increased. Lacking any clear mandate for planning, both federal and state governments tried to make marginal or incremental changes by a succession of actions that bore no clear relation to each other, lacked consistent data for planning, and were driven by incompatible demands to save money and expand both quality and quantity of care. In this situation, for-profit and nonprofit boundaries began to blur, and nursing homes and hospitals were nimble and imaginative in changing their practices and in influencing public policies. Home care, with more but weaker voices, had least influence and was fragmented in its structure.

It has also become clearer to public officials in this decade that long-term home care needed attention on its merits and not as an afterthought to medical care. Two results at least are important: first, concepts and broad designs for long-term and for home care began to emerge (Pepper Commission 1990); and second, a number of important research and demonstration initiatives in home care were carried out although their full history has yet to be written.

The introduction of waivers into the Medicare and Medicaid programs may prove more significant both for the data produced and for the choices that could alleviate economic and political strains. Under the Health Care Finance Administration waiver program for Medicaid, introduced in 1981, states were able to experiment with flexible ways to deliver services to homes as well as in institutions. Obtaining a Medicaid waiver usually involved negotiations between state and federal officials to determine which federal rules would be relaxed to permit a state to do something outside the established rules and regulations. Waivers encouraged state innovations, which would provide evidence about outcomes of different plans and become the basis for future federal policy. Over time, these tested the capacity of states, on a decentralized basis in a federal system, to act constructively on problems previously believed to be dependent mainly on federal decision-making. A major objective was to increase flexibility in use of federal dollars to substitute at-home or day care for avoidable hospital and nursing home admissions, through freer state use of social and medical services. Another aim was to permit states to use some of the expected savings to expand services to still unprotected populations and to reduce the reliance on nursing homes. An expected consequence was the impetus the waiver movement gave to transfer even more authority to the states via block grants to be used by the states with modified federal monitoring and without advance permission.

By 1990 most states were involved in many experiments, but no conclusive picture of results is available. Numerous partial analyses have been performed, but few definitive answers have been provided to the question of whether flexibility in using Medicaid funds led to diverting patients to home care. Nursing home occupancy has declined, and more people receive care at home, but there is no clear causal connection proving that home-care benefits alone are the major factor in patients remaining at home. The interaction of service availability, patient's condition, family networks, and much more is accompanied by less quantified data about how people make their choices. Still, it is at least clear that giving state agencies significant flexibility in using funds does produce greater choice to the patient and family, as well as to public officials managing long-term disabilities (Coleman 1996; Kassner and Martin 1996; Newman and Enval 1995; and National Conference of State Legislatures 1997). The privately funded Intergovernmental Health Policy Project has begun systematic collection of information from fifty states. Yet changes are occurring so rapidly that data for one year are overtaken by changes in the next.

POLICIES AND PROGRAMS

The Pepper Commission's strong statement about long-term home care offers crucial general principles and a broad design, without having implementing details in place. It led to the Home Care Catastrophic bill of 1987, which proposed to cover aged and all adults with disability in a Medicare home-care program. The bill was defeated, but parts of it remained in the broader Catastrophic Health Care legislation of 1988. Although it extended the number of days for "intermittent home care," it still required some medical justification. Nevertheless, it was also a watershed of legislative effort to integrate medical and long-term social care in one legislative mandate (Pepper 1990).

The Clinton administration's 1994 health care reform plan proposed a small step in the form of $300,000,000 from federal resources for home- and community-based care to be administered by the states. This *was* strongly supported but failed along with the rest of the plan when the need to control medical costs captured the debate. Although the long-term-care component was not central to the failure of the Clinton proposal, it is fair to say that no systematic effort has been made subsequently to advance the long-term care component of the plan.

CHAPTER 2 ❊ *The Number and Diversity of Persons Needing Home Care*

*T*HE POPULATION that home care is concerned with is not easily counted. It includes individuals of all ages who have limitations in either mobility or self-care or both. The matter is further complicated by how we define home care. Some national data refer to long-term care and to home health care, both of which include medical, nursing, and social support services. Other data combine informal care at home given by resident family members, unpaid volunteer helpers, and paid caregivers. Because most financing and organizational planning depend on projections into the near future at least, the demographic trends of an aging population and the estimates about whether disability is increasing or simply being compressed into fewer years at the end of life must be taken into account.

Our primary purpose, however, is to concentrate on those who need social supports or personal assistance, in addition to or apart from medical treatment while living at home or in the community. We try to keep these distinctions in mind. We seek to identify the population likely to benefit from personal assistance at home as that translates into public policy and financing. The 1990 census reports over 13 million persons so limited who live outside institutions. We would add to this number all those in institutions who could live at home if assisted.

In this chapter we present several characteristics of the population that home care needs to address now and in the future. These are no longer the simple home helps once provided by family but now offered by formal agencies because of changes in family life and the aging of the population. Age and family are still part of the stereotype that governs popular thinking and therefore the kind of services that home care is expected to offer.

More important, the diversity of conditions and populations that constitute the arena for home care has in the past led to a proliferation of specialized programs and agencies. All efforts to fit home care into a coherent system for programs and policies and for public funding are influenced by this fact. Whether the confusing variety of agencies and the confusing distribution of resources among numerous medical, health, nursing, and social welfare agencies is the best way to meet diverse needs or whether some regrouping in the field is required depends in part on understanding the diversity of populations and needs involved.

Questions of Definition

Part of the difficulty lies in the ambiguity of such phrases as "long-term care," "home care," and "chronic disability," which are used by different agencies for different purposes as the basis for planning. For example, service agencies and payers each have their own criteria of eligibility for service, and these in turn are aggregated to define numbers in need or entitled to reimbursement. Medicaid, Medicare, private insurance companies, hospitals, nursing homes, visiting nurse associations, day-care centers, rehabilitation centers, centers for independent living, assisted living centers, and many other groups each define whom they will serve, and this choice is influenced in turn by the available sources of reimbursement (Boaz and Muller 1994).

The useful criteria for identifying instrumental activities of daily living as measures of functional disability are often determined by self-reporting by an individual or by the subjective perception of another. For medical purposes, *long-term* usually means a few days, weeks, or perhaps months—whatever time it takes to complete active treatment until a patient can be discharged from a hospital's roster of cases under care, as restored to a previous condition of relative well being, or as lying outside a medical institution's sphere of responsibility. But it also embraces persons with severe chronic conditions persisting indefinitely, for months or years or even a lifetime, and requiring active medical attention. The term also means long persisting dependency on help from others for reasons other than a clinical diagnosis—successive episodes, multiple conditions, or dependency for reasons other than any underlying disease. The definition of mental illness has expanded to include a variety of behaviors once considered dysfunction rather than illness that require "long-term" care.

Who Is Responsible? Different Systems

Primary or initial public responsibility of caring for people with disabling conditions is divided between two major service systems—medicine and welfare, the former mainly for the short-term "treatable" episodes and the latter for long-term conditions not likely to benefit from short-term or episodic therapy. A number of subsystems fall between these two, for example, nursing homes, chronic disease hospitals (once called hospitals for the incurable), rehabilitation centers, and public health agencies. Mental health has become a major subset of medicine, and new epidemic diseases such as AIDS and antibiotic-resistant tuberculosis have introduced a new time dimension for active medical treatment plus the problem of control of communicable diseases for those who care for the physically dependent.

Medicine is used by all classes of citizens at some time, able bodied or not, whereas welfare is perceived as needed by the dependent poor, hapless, or helpless. All rely, to different degrees, on therapeutic interventions and social supports. All deal with functional limitations and dependencies for psychological, social, or economic reasons and are backed by different degrees of respect in society and by personnel with different skills.

Both policy and programs are also divided by age; some programs serve only the elderly, others only those under 65, and some only children. Each group requires similar personal assistance as well as different medical or nursing specialty services. The boundary between formal and informal care may vary for some. Children are more likely to have a family, but not always and the family may consist of only one single parent. The elderly may have adult children nearby, but perhaps 20 percent have no family at all. For home care, a simple template is not sufficient. Until recently medical care was accepted as essential for all, and welfare a regrettable necessity to be controlled. Recently escalating costs have subjected both systems to public pressure to control expenses and responsibilities have shifted.

Boundaries of the Population at Risk

Recent research into the politics of policy making introduces this caution in using data: apparently objective numbers turn out to be selectively drawn from a variety of sources most favorable for a particular policy purpose. Data showing low initial costs often omit other data projecting very large costs a few years later. The data are not viewed as tainted, only targeted to achieve a desirable end (Berkowitz and Gratton 1997).

Several efforts have been made to use more exacting criteria than activities of daily living in order to estimate potential need or demand for home-care services. A forthcoming report will review all criteria proposed for eligibility in programs under consideration by Congress (Maslow and O'Keeffe 1998). One such comprehensive effort was developed by an advisory task force for the Con-

gressional Office of Technology Assessment. It was never acted upon or published because the office was dismantled by Congress before a report was completed. It proposed the following elements for a medical system:

1. Cause—the underlying medical condition

2. Impaired organs—physiological abnormalities or loss of organ function

3. Personal function—limitation in everyday functions such as personal care,
   walking, and short-term memory loss

4. Environmental interaction—limitation in ability to perform socially expected roles or tasks.

The 1990 census used this classification for self-reporting: "Because of a
health condition that has lasted 6 months or more, does this person have any
difficulty (a) going outside the home alone or (b) taking care of his or her own
personal needs?

The Risk Population

We suggest using an aggregate total of persons potentially constituting the home
care "market" drawn from the census. A conservative estimate is that 13.2 million persons over the age of 16 have long-term self-care or mobility problems.
A more generous estimate places the figure as high as 31 million over the age of
18 who have some limitation but who are not necessarily dependent on frequent
daily help from others.

Against this number, some 3,272,000 persons received help from 7,000 home-
care agencies in 1991. Of the more than 13 million handicapped persons, 11 million live at home; an estimated 75 percent of their care is provided by family or
uncompensated helpers. Because these estimates are general, we discuss next the
ways that various sources arrive at them. These figures do not include institutionalized persons with conditions no more severe than those of people who live
at home. These could well be included for future planning.

Various Estimates of the Risk Population

The Census Bureau concluded that, in the civilian noninstitutional population
16 years and older, 13.2 million had a long-term functional disability. Of these
7.2 million between the ages 16 and 64 had either mobility or self-care limitations; more narrowly, 5.3 million had functional limitations. Of the 5.9 million

over the age of 65, 20.1 percent had either self-care or mobility limitations and 3.5 million over the age of 65 had functional disabilities. At ages 16–64, 2.2 percent have mobility limits and 3.4 percent have self-care limits. At age 65 and over, 15.6 percent have mobility limits and 11.9 percent have self-care limits. Figure 1 illustrates the types and levels of care required by the total at-risk population (U.S. Bureau of Census 1995, 1996).

Although disability rates are higher among the elderly than they are among other adults, the majority of adults with disabilities are under 65 years of age. Among those with self-care limitations 60.3 percent are between the ages of 16 and 64 and 39.7 percent are 65 years of age and older.

Of all persons identified by available measures as needing long-term care, 42 percent are under the age of 65, but there are 3.3 million over the age of 85; of these 50 percent need help daily. Instead of an old population, there seems to be a possible bipolar distribution among younger and the very old, with a valley of functional limits in between (Statistical Abstracts 1994; HCFA 1995). The picture is further complicated by the special problem of the 31 percent of the younger disabled who are able to work outside the home. Of the disabled between the ages of 21 and 26 who graduate from high school, 34 percent are employed and many of them need some help with transportation and intermittent help with daily activities.

The severity of care needs is especially clear for the 100,000 minor children who can live with family but are dependent on advanced technologies. Ventilators, once limited to the hospital, can be provided at home but place new demands on the family. There are about 200,000 young adults with spinal cord injuries who live at home with substantial personal assistance and complementing health care.

The Medical Dimension for Social Home Care

Disabling conditions are distributed differently by age. For those age 18–24 mental retardation, mental illness, and orthopedic handicaps predominate. For adults age 45–69 major disabilities are due to arthritis, heart disease, hypertension, and circulatory problems. Since 1980 AIDS has become a major wasting illness with no cure yet at hand.

The severity of causal conditions and the specialty attention each may demand play a large role in decisions about home care. Since hospitals are so important a referral source for home care, attention is needed to the kinds of cases they pass on. While a comprehensive summary is not available, the issue is illuminated in the practice of one major home health care agency—the

Fɪɢ. 1. Personal Assistance in the long-term care continuum

Phase 1 Treatment, cure, or restored function. A few days or weeks.		**Medical care dominant** In medical institution (hospital or nursing) with medical-related health services and predominance of public funding.
Phase 2 Extended or sub-acute care. A few weeks or months.		**Active medical and ancillary care controls—** Delivered either in an institution or at home. Personal assistance a necessary component provided by either family or formal home care service. Limited financing available.
Phase 3 Long-term chronic or incapacitating conditions. Care needed for months or for life.		**Personal assistance in some form dominant—** Access to intermitent medical care as needed. Personal assistance by family, other informal means, or by a formal agency at home or in an institution. Financing limited, uncertain and fragmented.

◼ Medical   ◻ Personal Assistance

Community Medical Associates (CMA), who contract with hospitals to provide full coverage for the hard-to-manage medical cases. Although the sample is small, and not at all representative of anything except the CMA caseload, it is suggestive. CMA reports that spinal cord injuries (paraplegia and quadriplegia) made up 39 percent of their referrals, 92 percent living at home. Severe but stable and severe degenerative neurological diseases (cerebral palsy and multiple sclerosis) make up another 60 percent. These conditions all require substantial integrated nursing and personal assistance plus medical treatments and monitoring, all of which can be provided in a home setting at a cost that compares favorably with that of a hospital or in a fragmented system. Other conditions commonly encountered are cancer, advanced AIDS, Parkinson's and muscular dystrophy (Master et al. 1996).

Such conditions have recently become more important in a consideration of social home care versus home health care. It may help to list the functional and behavioral conditions that accompany some of these medical conditions, which can be well served by home care. Few home care services are quite ready for the behaviors they may encounter. Each condition may have its distinctive needs and character or may share much with others. Some people with disabilities are characterized by uncontrollable body and facial movements that can be frightening or vaguely threatening. For others, rigidity of limbs and progressive loss of function make help necessary to perform the most simple of human acts—transferring, toilet, dressing. Some conditions involve excruciating pain and the medications can have side effects as bad as the pain. For others there are problems of changing cognition or increasing deficit in vision and hearing, which cumulatively interfere with human interaction, and lead to misunderstandings and confusion.

❊ Cerebral palsy is a paralysis caused by a prenatal brain defect or injury during birth. It is characterized by involuntary body motions and difficulty in controlling voluntary muscles.

❊ Multiple sclerosis, chiefly among youth, is characterized by speech disturbances, poor muscle coordination, weakness caused by sclerotic brain and spinal patches.

❊ Cerebral vascular disease involves the cerebrum and its blood flow, which controls body movements and coordinates many mental actions.

❊ Parkinson's disease is a nerve disease with tremors, muscle rigidity, and slowness in movement and speech. It is progressive ending in immobility, but not necessarily loss of cognition.

❊ Muscular dystrophy is a progressive deterioration and wasting away of muscles.

❊ Arthritis, very widespread, is a disease of the joints leading, among other things, to loss of cartilage and extreme pain.

Other Variables: How Many Are Needed?

The subject remains difficult to simplify despite topological efforts; activities of daily living begin to define the boundaries of a social problem but do not by themselves clarify how disability translates into concrete public policies and programs. For example, the number and proportion of disabled who live at home or in the community greatly exceed the number in institutions. Information about the former is limited. Individuals with the identical medical condition are about as likely to live in the community as in a nursing home, so what explains the difference? Is it difference in social supports, in causative condition, or technology used? Or is it difference in the individual's motivation or energy level?

By various estimates there may be 6–10 million severely disabled persons living in the community but there are fewer than 2 million residential facility beds. The University of Minnesota estimated, from the U.S. Census in 1990, that 12.6 million persons of all ages needed community or institutional services. Nearly 4 percent were aged 0–17 and, at the other extreme, nearly 58 percent of those were over 65. This can be used as a rough starting point. Differences in family status, education, income, and coping capacity of the individual all play a part. Another factor is the response time with which social and institutional service systems make decisions. The temperament of an individual may be the most powerful element but is least understood. Ability, or energy, to cope with physical limitations and to function with much pain differs among individuals. Mental retardation, memory loss, and vision deficits affect coping capacity, especially for those who must live alone.

Mental illness, bizarre behavior, or addiction to drugs and alcohol all may play a part, but who is responsible for managing the dependency? Are these medical or social problems, and is their duration the only thing that they share of responsibility and financing between medicine and welfare when the required span of service may range from a few weeks to many years?

Because conditions also change over time, service may be constantly shifted back and forth and continuity of information as well as attention is lost.

Although two-thirds of disabled persons live with and are cared for at home by their families (this encourages reliance on the family for home care), studies also indicate that family care can drop as much as 50 percent after two serious hospitalizations (Eggert et al. 1977). And some patient behaviors are so unbearable that families cannot continue to provide the necessary help; Alzheimer's disease in late stages is one example. Late stages in Parkinson's disease can involve such heavy physical care to meet the personal bodily needs that a family member can no longer carry on. Should such circumstances affect the way we estimate the social responsibility of a community or a society for disabled persons? So we see that attention to supporting families and their needs becomes an unexpected responsibility of home care. And as individuals and their family caregivers move into very old age, feebleness also takes its toll on both patient and family. Are such situations to be classified in the potential home care population, in the projected institutional population, as cause for admission to a medical or nursing institution, Or as a reason to rethink the home care function and its financing and structure? (See Chap. 3.)

Other data illustrate the difficulty service and financing agencies have in sorting out medical and social responsibilities.

1. About 4 million children under age 18 years and 21.7 million adults age 18–64 are limited in some degree in performing some major life activities. About 400,000 children and 7.8 million adults under 65 are unable to perform some major activity necessary in daily life—bathing, eating, dressing, toilet, or transfer from bed to chair (*Statistical Abstract* 1994).

2. Using age-specific measures of activities of daily living limitations, surveys of those receiving benefits from Social Security Disability Insurance (SSDI) and the Supplementary Security Income (SSI) programs reveal that there are 2.1 million adults age 45–64 (4.4 percent of the population) and 450,000 (1.2 percent) of adults 18–44 who are limited in some way in performing activities associated with self-care. About 2 percent of all under the age 65 are severely limited in three of five major areas (DHHS 1990).

3. Of those age 15–64 with serious daily living limitations (or 2 percent of those under 65), 44 percent require personal assistance (25 percent of those with one limitation and 67 percent for those with 3 or more limitations; DHHS 1990). The help required includes help with dressing, bathing, transferring.

4. Thirty-one percent of persons age 15–64 who are limited in daily living need some help to maintain themselves in the community because of limitation in their ability to perform instrumental activities such as housework or travel outside the home. Twenty-one percent need help in preparing meals.

5. Despite disability, a significant proportion can work with some supportive aid. Of those who have disability but also work, 31 percent require some personal assistance.

6. Of young adults age 21–26 with disabilities who have graduated from high school, 34 percent are employed, but 43 percent are not employed 3 years after

graduation. The mentally retarded, those with multiple impairments, those with orthopedic problems, and those who are deaf or blind are especially vulnerable and limited in function.

7. About 100,000 children are dependent on advanced technologies such as ventilators to remain alive but can function with them.

8. Of some 200,000 individuals, mainly young adults, with severe spinal cord damage, 92 percent live in the community with personal assistance.

9. The disabling conditions vary by age. Among those age 18–24, mental retardation, mental illness, and orthopedic problems are major limiting conditions. For those age 45–69 the major difficulties are arthritis, heart disease, and hypertension or circulatory problems.

A definitive picture of the population at risk is not globally available, but the diversity gives some sense of the boundaries for concern and helps explain the proliferation of numerous specialty service, financing, and advocacy groups.

Obstacles Presented by Diversity in the Target Population

It will help to examine the problems of such a diverse population as a foundation for discussing in Chapter 10 the financing and service modalities for the aggregated target population (Burbridge 1993; Stone and Kemper 1989).

1. The number of persons involved in the long-term care conundrum is relatively small compared with the conventionally defined health system. For example, of nearly 30 million persons recorded for Medicare in 1991, only 2 million received home *health* services during active treatment (a ratio of 94 beneficiaries per 1000). Inpatient or outpatient hospital and other physician or medical services are reported for over 45 million persons at the rate of 1496 per 1000 enrollees in Medicare. The relatively small role filled by home care may be due to persistence of hospital staff practices under pressure to move patients quickly. A nursing facility may be seen as safest while home care is arranged; or it may be due to limitations in the funding criteria built into the law with a bias to use medical necessity as a protection against increased demand. Equally, it may be due to limitations in capacity or vision of home care agencies to elaborate or increase their roles in long-term care or to unexpected changes in family composition.

Medicaid reported for 1992 that 31,150,000 recipients made 44,364,000 medical visits (hospital inpatient or out, nursing homes, and physicians' offices). Home health was reported for 926,000 recipients. This suggests how easy it is for hospital, medical, and nursing home services to dominate services to the public and also the attention of voters and policy makers because of sheer volume. By comparison, home care is relatively small.

2. The problem of attention is further complicated because the relatively small number of long-term disabled are, in turn, further subdivided into numerous diagnostic subcategories, each of which demands its special pattern of medical and technological needs, access to its own complex of medical specialists, and different patterns of social support need as linked to health care. They also differ in family composition, age, income, and adequacy (or inadequacy) of insurance or public provision. How is this population, segmented as it is among separate categories each partially dependent on medical attention and partially on diverse and scattered social supports, to find a place or niche either in the medical system or outside of it?

3. The personnel involved are differently organized. Medical personnel are identified with their basic institution, the hospital. Social support personnel are divided among nurses, nursing aides, social workers, physiotherapists, and others whose professional organizations are less influential than are those in medicine. One is seen as more scientific and reliable; the other less scientific and less convincing.

4. The advocacy and constituency organizations for home care have a national presence but they are underfunded, less influential, and much more divided in their aims and purposes than are medical organizations.

5. Cultural changes have been shifting public understanding about what is a normal or socially acceptable way of functioning with disability—at home or in an institution. The long history of family responsibility for the disabled and the extensive current reliance of so high a proportion of the disabled on family care for help presents policy makers with a serious dilemma, especially in an era of fiscal and political limitations. The combination of these circumstances has made it difficult to forge a coherent approach to long-term and home care that can compete with the overwhelming presence of medical care commitments built up in the past. The numerous formulas to overcome these limitations have not yet bridged concepts about human needs and their translation into public policy realities.

6. Individuals also have an almost limitless range of adaptive potential. Individuals with similar disabilities are found in institutions and at home, some living alone. We lack simple guidelines about who needs what and when, so we fall back on judgments made by doctors (busier than ever), social workers, and families. But the professional services now have difficulty getting to know individuals well enough to make critical judgments in situations not at crisis or life threatening, so they rely on vague criteria or subjective judgments.

Identifying populations for attention then results in professional specializations and advocacy groups focused on narrow conditions, often defined by families of persons with specific conditions. They become the activists, raise funds for research and lobby. The sum of specialization is a widening range of medical specialists. Any one condition can invoke participation of several medical specialties in order to settle on a diagnosis and prescription and a plan of treatment as well as on a plan for care. Most now depend on advanced technologies. Public and private funding develops around such units of advocacy.

Have These Populations and Agencies Anything in Common?

Despite these obstacles, progress has been made. The two enduring characteristics describing the diversified target population are: (1) All these conditions have some root in medical care and the sciences involved in medicine. There have been some gains in prevention and treatment, for example, in treatment of spinal cord injuries, although the long-term disabilities still resist conquest of so many infectious and public health or viral or bacterial diseases. The medical system already is involved in the short-term aspects of these conditions and relies on other long-term facilities to relieve hospitals of longer and costly hospital use. (2) A slow accumulation of concepts and proposals about how to manage and care for long-term severe disability represents a slow evolution in constituency and advocacy ability to find a place for these conditions just when all medical and health and welfare services are under pressure to reform and redesign their programs and practices to fit changes in public economy, demography, and public expectations.

The field has relied on the concept of "a seamless web of services" as a mantra to secure access to many kinds of services—acute treatment, prevention, specialist and primary physician help, nursing care, rehabilitation, social and personal attendant care, hospitalization or nursing home—all with minimum eligibility barriers, few delays in access to services, and subsidy for costs that exceed the "average" individual's means. Advocates for home care extend their hopes to include suitable training for each of the special services potentially needed and protection against neglect and fraud.

The weak link in the "web" has been personal care services, which are not medical but which can be essential for the severely disabled between visits from or to a professional. How much of this is a family expected to cover, and who will if there is no family or if costs exceed family means?

All parts of long-term care share an interest in seeing to it that underdeveloped parts of the system are filled out even while protecting their several interests. But how? The various disability interest groups, in the 1994 debate over health care reform, did form a coalition to support $300,000,000 to develop home care. The coalition did not succeed in rallying its "troops at home" to support the entire reform package and so lost the small home-care segment it contained. This suggests that there was more interest in the acute medical part of the reform than in the small step to home care, and less attention to how to make home care a part of an integrated medical system.

We discuss in our conclusions (Chapter 12) some approaches to the next stage in home-care evolution, stages that will involve a major rethinking in concept, strategy, and structure for home care to emerge as a system able to survive in the competitive world of the late 1990s—and more important, a system better able to deal with the contradictions in fitting together services to the range of populations potentially encompassed by home care while policies, funding, and agencies of all kinds are going through a time of continuous review. The following chapters analyze major factors in the movement to develop a viable system.

CHAPTER 3 ❋ *Family Roles in Providing Personal Assistance*

$\mathcal{F}$AMILIES ARE and will continue to be the major providers of long-term personal assistance for functionally disabled members. Family roles providing personal assistance are an aspect of the mutual aid that is fundamental to family life, reflected in the division of labor through which members assume complementary roles that sustain and further the social unit. Some of the roles that are performed on behalf of the functionally disabled are simply a continuation of roles that were already in place within the family prior to the onset of the disability. Other roles may have to be assumed in order to meet new conditions (Moen, Robison, and Fields 1994).

It is common to find that one member of a couple routinely performs certain household tasks even though the partner may be fully capable of performing that same task. (Sometimes a member fails to learn to perform some household tasks because the other routinely assumes the responsibility.) The roles that women often perform in meal preparation and men perform in home maintenance are good examples. Similarly, adult children may help older parents in such matters as preparing meals, providing rides, and maintaining the household even though the parents, strictly speaking, are capable of performing these tasks independently.

Households have varying histories in their use of paid services, as well. Patterns for using paid services differ widely in terms of circumstances reflecting family composition, financial resources, geographic location, social class, and subculture. For example, it is common for single mothers to pay for child care while they work. Some middle-class families with young children pay for child care to enable the a parent to get away for a short period of time or for a vacation. Depending on their circumstance, individuals and families routinely pay for personal services such as hair and nail treatments, local transportation, house cleaning, yard maintenance, tax preparation, and other aspects of domestic life.

Major normative questions with vast policy implications are: How much of the needed personal assistance should be provided by family members? And how should the responsibility for informal caregiving be divided among close relatives? To what extent should the functionally disabled and their family caregivers be expected to co-reside together or in close proximity to facilitate caregiving? To what extent should relatives be expected to modify their life patterns to accommodate caregiving demands? Some of the major public policy questions surrounding long-term care implicitly involve the manner in which publicly subsidized long-term-care services should complement the help provided by families (Beland 1984; Doty 1986).

This chapter examines the sources of personal assistance, the variety of forms it takes in relation to levels of functional disability, the limits on families as caregivers, and the future of caregiving.

Sources of Informal Personal Assistance

In the case of the elderly with disabilities, spouses and adult children are the major sources of informal care. If a spouse is available, the primary caregiver for the elderly disabled tends to be the spouse. The 1984 National Long-Term Care Survey revealed that 60 percent of primary caregivers to older people were wives usually caring for their husbands. Of these wives who were primary caregivers, 73 percent were aged 65 or over (Hooyman and Kiyak 1993). For children with developmental disabilities, parents are the major sources of personal assistance.

Women are the major providers of informal long-term care. Nearly 75 percent of all caregivers are women, and caregiving daughters outnumber caregiving sons three to one (Brakman 1994). Older men, however, are as likely as older women to be involved in caregiving. The Commonwealth Fund Productive Aging Survey of a representative sample of the noninstitutionalized population 55 years of age and older found that approximately 30 percent of both men and women reported that they were active in providing help to the sick and disabled. But two-thirds of the help to the sick and disabled was reported by women. The discrepancy is attributable to the greater longevity of women (Caro and Bass 1995).

Even when spouses are not considered, informal caregiving for the elderly tends to be provided by middle-age and older people. A study of caregiving by adult children between 45 and 64 years of age found that those between 45 and 54 were more affected by caregiving responsibilities than were older respondents. Among those in the 45–54 age group, 17 percent had a disabled older parent (Cantor 1992).

A significant proportion of potential informal caregivers of the functionally disabled elderly are themselves older: approximately 25 percent are between the ages of 55 and 64 and approximately 7 percent are 65 and older (Stone and Kemper 1989). Time given to informal help is sensitive to the extent of self-care deficits. Kemper (1992), for example, drawing upon data from the Channeling demonstrations, estimated the effects of adult daily living deficits upon hours of informal care per week, controlling for a set of other variables. He distinguished between resident informal care and visiting informal care. The response to increasing daily living deficits was particularly strong in the case of resident informal caregivers. When informal caregivers were visitors, the estimated effect of five daily living deficits was an increase of 7.7 hours of care per week. But when the informal caregivers resided with the care recipient, the number of hours of informal care per week was 37 hours greater than when there were no daily living deficits (Kemper 1992). The sensitivity of residence to hours of informal caregiving was particularly great when care recipients had three or more daily living disabilities.

Formal and informal care are largely complementary. When formal services are present, informal caregivers also tend to be involved. Only 5.5 percent of long-term care recipients who reside in the community receive help exclusively from formal services; 20.6 percent receive a combination of formal and informal help (Callahan 1996).

When care recipients and informal caregivers reside together, informal care has been found to be more sensitive to the extent of self-care deficits than formal care. Analyzing data from the Channeling demonstration, Kemper (1992) found a stronger relationship between the number of deficits for older people and hours per week for informal help than he did for formal help (Table 1). The increases in hours of formal help that were associated with increases in deficits were similar to those reported for visiting informal care; for those with five deficits, the amount of formal care was estimated to require 10 hours per week more than for those with no deficits. The visiting informal care for those with five deficit was estimated to require 8 hours per week more; as indicated above, the estimated amount for resident informal caregivers was 37 hours per week.

In many respects, informal care is often superior to formal care (Litwak 1985). Family members can be highly flexible in the forms of assistance they provide; they can be sensitive to the preferences of care recipients to subtle aspects of providing care; and they can readily combine companionship and emotional support with the performance of caregiving tasks. Informal care is particularly advantageous when caregivers and recipients reside together or nearby.

In the case of certain physically demanding tasks, formal services may be

TABLE 1. Estimated Total Effects of ADL Disability on Hours of Care per Week

ADL Disabilities	Formal Care	Visiting Informal Care	Resident Informal Care	Total
One	4.6	3.1	9.2	16.9
Two	5	2.9	7.8	15.7
Three	7.2	3.1	20.8	31.1
Four	8	5.3	30	43.3
Five	9.8	7.7	37.2	54.7

Source: Adapted from Kemper (1992).

Note: Based on Channeling Demonstration data; estimates are drawn from a multiple regression analysis that controlled for a number of other variables.

required. When the care recipient is heavy and needs help with transferring, for example, formal providers should have the physical strength that a family member may lack. Formal caregivers may also be better prepared to perform certain heavy housekeeping tasks. Formal services are better able to substitute for informal help with tasks that are readily defined, needed only intermittently, and lend themselves to scheduling, for example, laundry, house cleaning, and yard work.

When paid services are introduced, they may provide informal caregivers with occasional or extensive relief from tasks done previously or with tasks that were neglected, such as heavy housework or certain yard work. Family members, therefore, tend to continue to remain active but may shift their emphasis to other kinds of tasks.

Families may be flawed providers of long-term care. They may, for example, withhold or delay providing care. Abuse and neglect of the elderly by relatives is widespread enough to attract persistent professional attention (Pillemer and Wolf 1986). In some cases, family members may provide care but demonstrate a resentment of their obligation. In these cases, formal services may be a welcome replacement for unsatisfactory informal care.

Even when care is willingly provided by family members, recipients may be troubled by their dependence upon relatives and their inability to reciprocate adequately. Care recipients may strongly prefer a more autonomous position in which they can select their own providers of personal assistance. In some situations, then, access to formal services may "liberate" the care recipient. A preference for control over sources of personal assistance and independence from family caregiving is well established among the adult disabled. Current cohorts of older people with disabilities appear to be more accepting of care provided by family members and less insistent on formal care.

Family roles in providing personal assistance can be affected greatly by type of housing and household composition. Consider the situation of a hypothetical older retired married couple living in a suburban single family home. The closest adult child lives two to three miles away. Prior to the onset of the disability, the couple was largely self-sufficient in maintaining the household. In addition to caring for themselves, the couple maintained their home and property. They have been largely self-sufficient in household cleaning, routine maintenance (e.g., replacing light bulbs, washing windows, and doing yard work). Responsibility for household tasks was divided according to traditional gender roles: the wife carried major responsibility for food shopping, meal preparation, and light housekeeping. The husband carried responsibility for payment of bills, routine home maintenance, and shopping associated with maintenance. Prior to the onset of disability, each was self-sufficient in addressing daily living needs and the household was functioning smoothly.

The husband has a stroke that leaves him with a loss of physical mobility, loss of ability to write, and some speech loss. His wife is likely in the first instance to assume responsibility for the husband's personal assistance requirements and continue her household duties. She is likely to have much more driving to do. In addition to driving for shopping purposes, she provides substantial transportation for her husband. How she deals with the household matters previously performed by her husband is less certain. If her husband previously took care of all family finances, she may be challenged to learn how to do it. In families with more financial resources, household finances are likely to be more complicated, but more affluent families are in a better position to hire professional help to assist with finances. Certain maintenance may be taken care of less diligently. An adult son or daughter may help with some of it. The couple may pay to have certain work done that they previously did themselves. They may pay to have yard work done. They may more readily call in a plumbing service to take care of minor plumbing problems. If the husband's personal assistance requirements are great, the wife is less likely to be able to perform all of the household tasks that she previously performed.

If a married woman develops a serious disability and her husband assumes primary responsibility for her personal assistance, he must also take on the household responsibilities formerly carried by his wife such as food shopping, meal preparation, and light housekeeping. If he has not been involved in performing these tasks, he may have a good deal to learn before he can handle them competently. He is likely to be driving a good deal more for shopping and to provide transportation for his wife. He may be challenged to carry out all of these responsibilities adequately. His ability to carry out some his previous responsibilities such as household maintenance may be reduced.

The situation is likely to be much less complicated if the couple is living in an apartment in which they have no responsibilities for building or property maintenance. If they live close to shopping and health care providers, the challenge of managing transportation is also likely to be substantially diminished.

Residential proximity of adult offspring is particularly important for the elderly disabled who are widowed, divorced, or separated. The situation of the disabled who live in the same household as adult offspring or other relatives is very different from that of the disabled who live alone at some distance from family. Particularly challenging is the situation of the disabled person who lives alone in a single-family house.

The ability of family members to assist with personal care and household matters that require regular attention is obviously affected greatly by residential proximity. Extensive participation is possible only when a relative and the disabled person live in the same household or nearby. (The importance of co-residence for intensity of informal caregiving is demonstrated in Table 1). In some cases the onset of disability or even the anticipation of disability triggers a move to achieve residential proximity that will facilitate extensive informal caregiving. In some of these cases, one or both move to a common residence. In other cases, the move brings the caregiver and recipient into greater physical proximity. Long visits may also be arranged to permit extensive temporary informal caregiving. The preference for independence in residence remains strong, but an elder's need for personal assistance may overcome the reluctance of both a parent and an adult son or daughter to share a residence.

Informal assistance in a household often has a long history that precedes the personal assistance that is provided after the onset of disability. As indicated above, one member of a couple routinely performs certain household tasks even though the partner may be fully capable of performing those tasks. (Sometimes a member fails to learn to perform some household tasks because the other routinely assumes the responsibility.) The roles that women often play in meal preparation and men play in home maintenance are good examples. Similarly, adult children may help parents in such matters as preparing meals, providing rides, and maintaining the household even though parents, strictly speaking, are capable of performing these tasks independently. Informal caregivers may increase the frequency of these forms of assistance as recipients age.

Prior to the onset of a disability, households also have varying histories in their use of paid services. These patterns are perhaps best understood among middle-class populations that can afford to pay for some services. Middle-class families, for example, are accustomed to hiring babysitters for young children to enable parents to get away for short periods of time. When children are young, families also frequently use formal child-care services to permit parents to participate in the labor force.

Access to formal services can also be a factor in selecting a residence. Some choose a rental unit or purchase a condominium that comes with extensive building services that include all aspects of exterior maintenance. Maids are now relatively uncommon, but in upper-middle-class households the use of house-cleaning services is relatively common. In some households, the consumption of foods prepared elsewhere is common. Some of those living in single family homes make regular use of paid help to take care of most aspects of exterior maintenance throughout the year.

For households that have purchased services regularly, the introduction of services to address personal assistance needs arising from disability is an incremental step. Because of their experience in using formal services to assist the household, they are likely to make the transition readily. Those with a history of using formal services are likely to know how to locate service resources, negotiate prices, establish their expectations regarding service delivery, and resolve problems with service delivery.

Other households have little or no history in the use of paid services performed within the household. Some have a long established pattern in which all household work is done on an unpaid basis. Even ambitious home improvement work is done on a do-it-yourself basis or through the unpaid help of friends or relatives. For these households, the introduction of paid help represents a significant transition. Household members may experience substantial difficulties in locating paid help, negotiating terms, and supervising the work. Household members may also be challenged to adjust to the presence of strangers in the household, especially if they are present for long periods of time on a sustained basis. At issue are both privacy and autonomy. Privacy is of particular concern when personal assistance is needed and when residential quarters are small. Autonomy is of concern to the degree that the care recipient is required or feels pressure to comply with constraints associated with the provider of formal care. The care recipient, for example, may need to accept the scheduling options offered by the care provider. The care recipient may have limited choice regarding the times when the provider is available. Much more subtle are accommodations that a care recipient may accept in the manner in which a formal provider performs various tasks. A care recipient may have very well established routines for addressing daily living tasks. While the care recipient may expect that a formal service provider will respect basic aspects of these routines, the care recipient must be prepared to accept some compromises. There may be differences, for example, in the manner in which food is prepared and served or in the manner in which house cleaning is done. Contributing to tension over the manner in which tasks are performed and even patterns of interaction are differences between care providers and care recipients in social class, race, and ethnicity. Almost half of home-care workers, for example, are foreign born (Chichin 1989). Consumers clearly vary in the degree to which they attach importance to these matters. For some individuals, retaining control over the manner in which household tasks are performed is important. The desire for control may lead to refusal to accept much-needed personal assistance.

Explaining Family Caregiving

Providing long-term care on a sustained basis is inherently challenging. As a form of paid work, long-term care is widely considered to be relatively unattractive. Fewer still are willing as volunteers to provide long-term care to strangers on a continuing basis. Yet, families provide the vast majority of long-term care. A number of studies have estimated that approximately 80 percent of the long-term care in the United States is provided by families (Biaggi 1980; Brody 1981; U.S. Senate Special Committee on Aging 1992). The fact that families provide the majority of long-term care suggests that the forces propelling the extensive family role must be powerful.

The expectation that marriage partners will care for one another is built into the institution of marriage. (Traditional vows, for example, refer explicitly to the obligations that partners assume for one another in times of sickness.) Expectations of responsibility for providing care extend from married couples to their children. The survival and development of infants is dependent on the care and nurturing provided by parents. In the vast majority of cases, parents fully understand and freely accept these responsibilities. In successful families, children acquire a strong loyalty to parents and siblings. Children learn to perform tasks needed by other family members and the household as a whole. Children develop a commitment to assist their parents out of affection, obligation, or a combination of the two. In some Asian societies in which family bonds are particularly strong, the obligation of adult children to their aging parents is an important aspect of filial piety (see, for example, Sung 1994).

While the responsibility of families to provide personal assistance is consistent across cultures, the strength of the obligation may vary substantially. The form that assistance is expected to take, the specific obligations of family members, the acceptability of using formal services to complement informal care may vary from one culture to another.

The strong role that families play in providing long-term care is explained, then, in part by the expectations built into marriage. Family members may experience an obligation to help, see helping as an opportunity to show affection, see helping as a way of reciprocating for help received in the past, or a combination of these (Rossi and Rossi 1990).

For older people, informal caregiving can also provide an important opportunity to assume a meaningful social role (Doty and Miller 1993). As a society we undervalue the productive capacity of older people. Many older people seek productive engagement (Caro and Bass 1995). Opportunities, particularly in paid employment, are very limited for them. For some, informal caregiving provides a welcome opportunity to be a contributing member of society.

Caregiving may also be propelled by guilt or fear of guilt. Family members may seek to avoid guilt resulting from the failure to meet the obligation to help or guilt from failure to reciprocate for help previously received. Spouses and adult offspring are sensitive to the fact that older people experiencing disabilities prefer informal assistance (Stoller and Cutler 1993).

Contributing to the strong role of families in providing personal assistance is the fact that the elderly disabled tend prefer to receive personal assistance at home. The preference for home care stems from negative attitudes toward nursing homes even though the quality of care in many nursing homes is good (Hatch and Franken 1984). "The nursing home, with its lack of independent quarters and highly structured medical-like environment, is the residence of 'last resort'" (Pynoos and Golant 1995, 303).

The disabled may prefer to be self-sufficient; they may also be reluctant to make demands on relatives. (Many do not want to be a burden on others.) The alternatives of finding an acceptable stranger to provide help, the loss of privacy associated with the presence of a stranger in the household, and the prospect of having to pay for help out of meager means may contribute to the preference for a family member to be the source of help.

The preference of older people to live near their children but apart from them illustrates the value that they attach to independence. "The majority of persons age 65 and over live near their children, sharing a social life but not their homes. Most elderly state that they prefer not to live with their children, generally for reasons of privacy and a sense of autonomy" (Hooyman and Kiyak 1993, 275).

Limits of Families as Personal Assistance Providers

Like other advanced societies, the United States is committed to furthering individual rights. We are committed to the principle that everyone has a right to certain individual development. In fact, the rights of the disabled furthered by the Americans for Disabilities Act are based upon principles of universal individual rights. The aim of the legislation is to assure that the disabled experience the same rights as those enjoyed by the majority to live and work in the community (Callahan 1996).

Family obligations are sometimes challenged by individual rights. Our society supports the right of individuals to leave unsatisfactory marriages. Our society is also sympathetic to those who are severely constrained in leading a normal life because of caregiving obligations. Individual rights of caregivers, therefore, may provide the basis for establishing limits to caregiving obligations.

Some critics have raised concern that personal assistance in the United States relies too much on the efforts of informal caregivers. Researchers have found evidence showing that in some cases caregiving contributes to mental distress or deterioration in physical health. (For a review of this extensive literature, see Stern 1995.) The research shows that the life patterns of caregivers are also sometimes adversely affected by caregiving. In some cases, caregiving interferes with paid employment. In other cases, for example, caregiving adversely affects geographical location; caregivers move to be with the care recipient or they are prevented from moving to a preferred part of the country.

Research evidence regarding adverse effects of caregiving is mixed. A minority of caregivers report burden. As might be expected, the more severe the disability of the care recipient, the more likely is the caregiver to report burden. Family members caring for those with cognitive deficits are also more likely to report burden than those caring for a relative with physical limitations alone. Surprisingly, the amount of time that caregivers report spending on caregiving is not consistently associated with burden. The high proportion of nursing home residents with cognitive deficits can be interpreted as a reflection of the difficulties that informal providers experience when they care for this population themselves.

Research evidence is available also showing positive effects of caregiving. Doty and Miller (1993) summarizes literature showing that caregivers tend to interpret their experiences positively. Motenko (1989) found that in relationships where there was strong love and affection between the caregiver and care recipient, effects of the experience on caregivers was more likely to be positive. In fact, burden and satisfaction sometimes go hand in hand because caregivers derive satisfaction from their ability to rise to a challenge. In the Common-wealth Fund's Productive Aging study of a representative sample of the nonin-stitutionalized population of those 55 years of age and older, 31 percent of the respondents reported that they were caring for the sick and disabled. Of these, 12 percent indicated that they were simultaneously experiencing heavy or mod-erate burden and deriving a great deal of satisfaction from their caregiving (Caro and Bass 1992). Alley (1988) also found caregiving to be both a positive and neg-ative experience for some.

The research evidence provides some support both for advocates of inter-ventions that would provide greater relief to families and for those who see lim-ited need for interventions to assist caregivers. The evidence indicates that only a minority of caregivers have complaints; if assistance were offered to care-givers, then, only a minority might seek to take advantage. In an evaluation study of a respite demonstration Lawton, Brody, and Saperstein (1989) found that only half of the families eligible for the respite services took advantage of the opportunity. In judging the merit of an intervention to assist caregivers, it is not clear how much response should be expected. We should anticipate that in a substantial proportion of intense caregiving situations, caregivers will pass up opportunities for assistance. Their reluctance to accept services may reflect a preference to provide care personally, reservations about the assistance that is available, and objections on the part of the care recipient.

Sweden provides unexpected evidence of the limited role of formal services in complementing informal care. Sweden is well known for its highly developed long-term care service system that provides a wide range of subsidized personal assistance options to the elderly. But recent research in Sweden has shown that in spite of the well-developed formal service system, nearly 75 percent of the hours of help provided to the elderly come from informal sources. Only among the very old is the amount of formal care equal to the amount of informal care (Johansson and Thorslund 1993). The predominance of informal long-term care in Sweden is instructive of the strong preferences of care recipients and family members for informal long-term care (Lesemann and Martin 1993).

The implications of efforts to expand formal home- and community-based long-term care in the United States for informal caregiving should be kept in perspective. Expansion of formal services tends not to decrease informal care-giving. Expansion of formal services is more likely to redistribute the types of assistance provided by informal caregivers. Expanded formal services tend to increase the assistance received by the disabled and enable informal caregivers to place greater emphasis on more expressive forms of assistance. Because long-term care in the United States is so heavily weighted toward informal care, an increase in formal services in the magnitude of 25 percent would be required to bring the percentage of share of informal care down from 80 percent to 75 percent.

Role of Families Clouds Prospects for Publicly Supported Personal Assistance

The high degree of involvement of informal caregivers has complicated the political debate about public support for home- and community-based long-term care. Public officials are most readily persuaded that public funding for home- and community-based care is justified when the care recipient has no informal caregivers. Some politicians have argued that long-term care is a family obligation. Their premise is that subsidized formal services would substitute for informal care when families are present. Although the research literature provides little evidence of substitution, some politicians remain skeptical. The path of least resistance for advocates for subsidized services is to emphasize personal assistance services for those without family members.

To the extent that advocates have sought public support for formal services that would provide relief to caregivers, their rationale has emphasized adverse effects of caregiving for informal caregivers. That rationale deserves reexamination. Should we have evidence that caregivers suffer adverse effects to mental or physical health or that their employment status is seriously jeopardized before more relief is offered at public expense? An alternate argument on relief for caregivers can be based on their rights as individuals. A case can be made, for example, that when self-care deficits and behavioral problems go beyond a threshold level, the care requirements of the disabled exceed the level that informal caregivers by themselves should be expected to absorb. In these cases, support should be offered to assure that alternatives to informal care are available. Public programs that offer assistance to families under these conditions would be judged successful if the resources were used on behalf of the disabled family member and if the life patterns of caregivers more closely approximated that of their peers.

A complicating factor in specifying a public obligation to provide relief to the efforts of informal caregivers is the capacity of informal systems to expand by involving multiple caregiving friends and relatives. In most instances, the majority of informal care is provided by a single individual. In many instances, however, other relatives can be identified who at least theoretically might participate significantly in providing care. A narrow interpretation of public responsibility is that relief should be offered to informal caregivers only as a last resort, that is, when there are no relatives who could reasonably be expected to provide relief to the primary informal caregiver. A more generous interpretation is that the participation of secondary informal caregivers should be encouraged but should remain voluntary. In effect, then, relief would be provided to primary caregivers at public expense when caregiving demands exceed a specified threshold.

The strategies employed by higher income families with personal assistance responsibilities deserve more attention. Particularly instructive are the actions by these families when they live in communities with well-developed service options for the self-pay market. Patterns of purchasing services by those who can afford them offers insights into the way that formal services can complement informal care when consumers have options and financial barriers are not important. Of interest are the types of service modalities selected and the duration of their use; also of interest are consumer opinions about these services. Concerns about loss of privacy and reservations about the skills of personal assistants, for example, may be important factors limiting the use of paid services.

The Future of Family Caregiving

Looking forward to the next twenty-five years, we see that families will remain the major providers of long-term care. At the same time, some important shifts may occur in the roles of family members as caregivers.

The most important single factor for the future of informal caregiving is the growth of the older population with disabilities. As those in the baby boom generation reach old age, the number of older people with disabilities will increase substantially. The major increase, however, will take place more than twenty-five years from now, when the baby boomers begin to reach 75 years of age. The need for long-term care will be affected by changes in disability rates among the elderly. If the period of disability in late life is indeed compressed, the proportion of older people requiring long-term care will decline somewhat.

A key factor for informal caregiving will be the extent to which the elderly disabled will have spouses. Among the factors that will affect the potential availability of spouses will be marital status of those entering old age and survival rates in married couples. The higher mortality rates experienced by men has accounted for the large numbers of older women with disabilities and without a husband to care for them. Recent increases in survival rates among men have resulted in a slight reduction in the age discrepancy in the survival rates between men and women. But because of higher divorce rates, more men and women enter old age without a spouse. As a result, little overall change can be expected in the extent to which older men and women will have a spouse available as a potential caregiver (Treas 1995).

Another major question is the extent to which the elderly with disabilities will have adult offspring who are potential caregivers. Long-term declines in family size imply that the number of potential caregiving children is likely to diminish. One recent study projected that for the elderly, the average number of living children will decline from 2.9 in 1990 to 1.9 in 2030 (Tennstedt, Crawford, and McKinlay, 1993b). Increasing rates of geographic mobility, however, invite questions about the extent to which adult children will live close enough to their parents with disabilities to play a significant caregiving role.

The tendency for older people to survive longer has implications for the age of their informal caregivers. For the cohorts that tended to marry and have children relatively early in life, delayed onset of late-life disabilities means that their adult offspring will tend to be older when they may be asked to provide informal long-term care. Increasingly, we can expect that caregiving sons and daughters will themselves be older people.

Future labor force participation patterns will have implications for the ability of informal caregivers to provide extensive care. At present, men are typically out of the labor force by age 62 and women tend to stop working even earlier. The age at which men leave the workforce has dropped substantially since World War II but has stabilized in recent years. Increasingly, women's labor force participation will tend to approximate that of men. In midlife, women will typically be in the work force and they will remain in the labor force as long as do men; they will not be available to make caregiving their primary activity. However, even if the labor force participation of both men and women should increase, many of the young elderly, that is, those between 55 and 65 years of age, will be out of the workforce. The increased involvement of adult women with the work place will have important implications for care of children and young adults with severe disabling conditions. Because of their employment commitments, parents will tend to be less available to provide care during normal working hours.

More speculative are questions about the continuing willingness of family members to perform extensive roles in long-term care. Will we see a shift in the willingness of family members to devote themselves to personal assistance? The widespread patterns of serial marriages may have important implications for the willingness of adult children to provide care (Binstock, Cluff, and von Mering 1996). To what extent, for example, will adult offspring be willing to provide extensive care to a parent who was absent during most of their childhood? To what extent will adult children be available to provide care to a stepparent? We suspect that less durable marriages will lead to a weakening of family responsibility for personal assistance of aging parents. Cultural trends that emphasize the rights of individuals will also be pertinent. An important societal theme is the increased emphasis placed upon the right of individuals to pursue their fulfillment. The implication is diminished responsibility to other institutions. The pursuit of individual rights may mean a reduced willingness of family members to provide personal assistance.

The increasing emphasis on individual rights also has implications for the adult disabled. For them, that includes a right to live an adult life that is independent of their parents. As the adult disabled are successful in establishing their right to a residence and personal assistance services apart from their parents, they are implicitly relieving their parents of significant caregiving responsibilities.

Reduced differentiation between male and female roles has implications for the future of informal caregiving. With the increased involvement of men in the care of their children and greater participation in household roles such as shopping, meal preparation, and laundry, men are likely to have greater receptivity to the household chores and personal assistance involved in providing personal assistance. The increasing involvement of women in home maintenance and household finances will assure that women will more readily be able to assume those responsibilities if necessary. But the opening of a wider range of opportunities may have long-term implications for the willingness of women to perform extensive caregiving roles. Even if women have been adding new roles without diminishing in their performance of more traditional roles, their willingness to perform multiple roles at a high level of intensity may diminish over time. If in the future, adult daughters are less willing to serve as primary caregivers to an aging parent, it is not at all clear that adult sons will be more willing to do so than they have in the past.

An important question for the future is how informal care will be affected by the expanding interest in assisted-living facilities among those who can afford to pay for their own care. Significant numbers of middle-class people find assisted living an attractive compromise that offers an efficient setting for the delivery of personal assistance services while it enables the disabled to retain substantial independence. The assisted-living option has complex implications for couples when one requires extensive personal assistance and the spouse is independent. The assisted-living facility offers the disabled person necessary personal assistance services. For the spouse, the move to assisted living means reduced responsibilities both for household maintenance and long-term care.

The relocation may, however, involve leaving a residence to which the couple has strong attachments. Furthermore, for the spouse, life in the group residence is likely to involve some unwelcome restrictions on independence. In the group residence, the spouse's involvement in personal assistance will continue, but the responsibilities for personal assistance services are shared. For some couples in this situation, the introduction of more extensive formal home care may be a more attractive option than a move to assisted living. A strong formal home-care package may be sufficient to provide significant relief to the informal care-giver and yet allow the informal caregiver to enjoy the independence associated with living at home.

Assisted living also has interesting implications for adult offspring who are primary caregivers. An assisted-living facility may be attractive to an adult child because the scope of personal assistance required by an aging parent is beyond what the son or daughter is able to provide. The adult child may have a major role in selecting the assisted-living facility and in monitoring services. The adult child's responsibility for day-to-day personal assistance services may be eliminated entirely by the parent's move to an assisted-living facility. The adult child may remain in close contact by visiting frequently and assisting with special needs that arise intermittently like shopping and transportation. Families that can afford to do so are often likely to find this option attractive. It relieves adult children of the need to provide day-to-day personal assistance services, and it permits the disabled parent to avoid being a burden to children. Further, if the assisted-living facility is close enough, it permits substantial personal contact and involvement with intermittent needs and expressive activities.

A question that is pertinent for the future whether older people with disabilities will demand greater independence from their adult children. Future generations of older people may be less willing to accept extensive help from their adult children. In the future, older parents may expect less of their adult children and may be more reluctant to impose upon them. Increasingly, they may prefer to pay for any personal assistance they need if they can afford to do so or use any subsidized services that may be available to them.

Of interest for the future also is informal care in old age for those whose need for personal assistance began relatively early in life. Because life expectancies for the disabled have improved dramatically, many can now expect to live to an old age. This group is less likely than the population as a whole to have married and to have adult children in old age. Their primary informal caregivers are likely to have been their parents. When they outlive their parents, siblings are the most likely sources of informal care. Increasingly, the adult disabled have a history of extensive use of formal services. For many, the use of formal services was important in establishing independence from parents. For those with disabilities who have established independence from parents relatively early in life by using formal personal assistance services in their own residences, we expect that the pattern of limited use of informal care will continue as they grow old.

At present, informal caregivers of the elderly are not a vocal political force asking for relief at public expense. For the most part, if caregivers of the elderly come together at all, they do so in support groups where they seek advice and assurance. Collectively, caregivers for the elderly have not spoken out forcefully either for subsidized services that would provide them with relief or for some financial compensation.

Alzheimer's disease caregivers have organized successfully but not as effective advocates for extensive publicly funded respite services. The Alzheimer's Association has been an effective advocate for the allocation of federal funds for research to understand the causes of the disease. The reluctance to lobby for relief to caregivers may stem from the fact that Alzheimer's disease strikes across the political spectrum. Significant numbers of Alzheimer's disease activists may be lukewarm to publicly subsidized efforts to assist caregivers because of a general aversion to new tax-supported domestic assistance programs of any kind.

Families with adult children with developmental disabilities are another exception. In some states, organizations representing these parents have spoken out forcefully regarding the needs for improved group home options for their children and for family supports. In some states in recent years, significant measures have been adopted to provide support to family caregivers. The greater willingness of families of children with disabilities to organize politically may stem from differences in the duration of disability. For children who are born with significant disabilities or who acquire them in early life, it is apparent to families that the condition is long-term. In these cases, families have strong reason to seek long-term measures for dealing with the consequences of disability. Contemporary thinking has also emphasized the right of these children to approximate normal lives. Significant interventions at public expense are almost always needed if that is to be accomplished. In the case of older people who receive extensive informal care after they acquire disabilities late in life, the duration of their need for extensive informal care is uncertain but often relatively brief. Caregivers who face the prospect of providing extensive care for six months to several years are perhaps less likely to mobilize politically than are the parents whose children have a whole life with a disability ahead of them.

A major question for the future is the extent to which long-term care will remain largely a family matter. We anticipate that over the years the interface between families and formal services in their relative responsibilities for long-term care will be more fully articulated. We expect that future generations of caregivers for the elderly will want to retain a strong hand but that they will also want to make greater use of formal services. We expect that future caregivers are more likely to insist on being case managers for their spouse or parent. We anticipate that those who can afford long-term care insurance will insist on policies that include strong respite provisions. For those who are eligible for publicly subsidized home-care services, we anticipate much greater scrutiny of the circumstances in which the availability of informal providers of care may limit eligibility for formal services.

$\mathcal{T}$HE LABOR FORCE that home-care staff is drawn from is often viewed by the public as consisting primarily of unskilled workers performing relatively simple household tasks that in the past would have been taken care of by family members. This view may once have been accurate, but the situation today has become much more complicated. Medical care systems now discharge patients when they still require substantial help. At the same time, technology for delivering more complex care in the home has improved; this entails not only the coordination of visits by technical specialists but also integrated personal assistance. From the perspective of services at home—social home care—however, the paid personal care assistant is the basic staff upon which the system depends, after the family, and without which the intermittent visits by treatment specialists have limited effect.

The boundaries between the growing typologies are no more exact than the different levels of skill required. When is a brief periodic (weekly) visit by a nurse sufficient and what help is needed in between? What is the relationship between the authority of the skilled nurse during her or his visit and that of the personal aide? In most cases it is assumed that a personal aide should have some special experience or training, but for social home care, the expectations for the personal care staff remain limited. The house visits of skilled professionals are curtailed but expectations about their help is very high.

Failure to deal with the complexity of home care staffing and how it is financed constitutes one of the handicaps the field needs to address. Home care may involve an array of staff ranging from trained nurses to home care aides to physical, occupational, respiratory, and speech therapists. They may also provide social work and nutritional care as well as laboratory, dental, optical, pharmacy, podiatry, and X-ray services, and tend to medical equipment and supplies. Home care services can be provided by the following professionals, paraprofessionals, and volunteers.

❋ Physicians visit patients in their homes to diagnose and treat illnesses just as they do in hospitals and private offices. They also work with families and home care providers to determine which services are needed by patients, which specialists are most suitable to render these services, and how often these services need to be provided. With this information, physicians routinely prescribe and oversee patient care plans.

❋ Registered nurses and licensed practical nurses provide skilled services that cannot be performed safely and effectively by nonprofessional personnel. Some of these services include injections and intravenous therapy, wound care, education on disease treatment and prevention, and patient assessments. Registered nurses may also provide case management services. Licensed practical nurses have one year of specialized training and are licensed to work under the supervision of registered nurses. The intricacy of a patient's medical condition and required course of treatment determine whether care should be provided by a registered nurse or can be provided by a licensed practical nurse.

❋ Physical therapists work to restore the mobility and strength of patients who are limited or disabled by physical injuries through the use of exercise, massage, and other methods. Physical therapists often alleviate pain and restore injured muscles with specialized equipment. They also teach patients and caregivers special techniques for walking and transfer.

❋ Social workers evaluate the social and emotional factors affecting ill and disabled individuals and provide counseling. They also help patients and their family members identify community resources. Social workers often serve as case managers when patients' conditions are so complex that professionals need to assess medical and supportive needs and coordinate a variety of services.

❋ Occupational therapists help individuals who have physical, developmental, social, or emotional problems that prevent them from performing the general activities of daily living. They instruct patients on using specialized rehabilitation techniques and equipment to improve their function in tasks such as eating, bathing, dressing, and basic household routines.

❋ Speech language pathologists work to develop and restore the speech of individuals with communication disorders; usually these disorders are the result of traumas such as surgery or stroke. Speech therapists also help retrain patients in breathing, swallowing, and muscle control.

❋ Dietitians provide counseling services to individuals who need professional dietary assessment and guidance to manage an illness or disability properly.

❋ Home care aides and home health aides assist patients with everyday activities such as getting in and out of bed, walking, bathing, toilet, and dressing. Some aides have received special training and are qualified to provide more complex services under the supervision of a nursing professional.

❋ Homemaker and chore workers perform light household duties such as laundry, meal preparation, general housekeeping, and shopping. Their services are directed at maintaining patient households rather than providing hands-on assistance with personal care.

❋ Companions provide companionship and comfort to individuals who, for medical and/or safety reasons, may not be left alone. Some companions may assist clients with household tasks, but most are limited to providing sitter services.

❋ Volunteers meet a variety of patient needs. The scope of a volunteer's services depends on his or her level of training and experience. Volunteer activities may include companionship, emotional support, counseling, and helping with personal care, paperwork, and transportation.

Work roles in home care and community-based long-term care can be viewed much more broadly than the positions of those who are directly involved in administering home care programs. The field also includes those who are extensively involved in designing, marketing, and administering claims for private long-term care insurance, in providing legal advice for estate planning to families concerned about long-term care costs, financial planners who help people save in anticipation of long-term care costs, architects who design residences to accommodate the disabled, hardware and software engineers who design assistive devices, planners and administrators of various community services such as home-delivered meals, out-of-home respite services, and specialized transportation that supports home care.

The two largest groups in the home care field are home care workers and case managers. Case managers are discussed in Chapter 11. This chapter covers home care workers who are variously called home aides, homemakers, chore workers, and, more recently, personal care assistants. They may live in or remain for several hours each day; some are nurses aides with some skill training. Their relationship to skilled health professional or paraprofessional staff who visit at intervals, such as registered nurses, physical and occupational therapists, physicians, as part of a medical care plan is considered again in Chapter 8. When the latter visit regularly, are they to be considered by the family as part of one home-care team either by contract or employment? Who is responsible, the home care agency or the other medical providers?

Size of the Home Care Labor Force

In 1993, home health care services reported 474,000 workers. In 1992, there were 347,000 workers identified as home health aides, projected to increase to 827,000 (a moderate projection) by 2005; 127,000 personal and home care aides are projected to increase to 293,000 by 2005. Some family members may be included. Nursing and personal care facilities in 1993 employed 1,615,000 nurses, aides, and attendants (up from 1,198,000 in 1985). Suzman and Manton estimated in 1992 a need for about 500,000 home health aides (see also Statistical Abstract 1994, tables 169, 639; Feldman 1988; Callahan 1996). Changes in the number of disabled or frail patients, in agency structures, in general labor market conditions, and, since the 1980s, in hospital admission and discharge policies and in third-party payment levels interact to influence changes in projected estimates.

Despite the sometimes unattractive nature of the work, the demand for aides and paraprofessional workers was projected to grow *by 600,000 for aides in institutions and by 475,000 for home care workers* between 1992 and 2005 (Silvestri 1993). This places the field among the top twelve growth occupations in the nation. Studies by Feldman (1988) predicted that the manpower situation could reach crisis proportions by 2002, when nine million elderly are expected to require 1.25 million aides of several types or three times the number employed in 1988. In addition physicians, nurses, social workers, laboratory workers, and others may be employed for temporary or intermittent or supervisory visits to the home. Health services, except hospitals, employed 5,521,000 in 1993 while home health services reported 474,000 employees of all kinds. Recently a few hospitals have begun to acquire or manage home care agencies for subacute posthospital care, complicating the issue of who is responsible for what care and for how long at home.

Social home care agencies confront specific problems of their own; the manpower pool upon which they rely also provides personal attendants for nursing homes, hospitals, and families using informal caregivers. The interrelationships between paid personal care provided in a home setting and health care services is considered in further detail in Chapter 8.

The Home Care Agencies

The home care agency infrastructure includes 7,000 home health care agencies and 1,000 hospice providers. These figures do not include some of the less easily defined social home care agencies or broker services with a fee for service counselling, which includes helping clients and families plan for their needs and then arranging to secure the agreed on services from other agencies (Statistical Abstract 1994, tables 194–195).

The reporting agencies in 1991 served 1,284,200 patients/clients on the survey day; in the year preceding the survey served 3,271,900. The latter figure suggests that much of the services were for the short-term not for long-term care. Eighty-five percent of the home health agencies are both Medicare- (which covers limited home care) and Medicaid-certified. Home care as an occupation is predicted to be one of the fastest growing in the next decade.

Home care agencies are at a disadvantage in competing for skilled workers against nursing home and other institutions, which can offer better pay, benefits, and security. The existence of willing unpaid family members also affects the demand for agency workers. For home care, nursing homes offer strong competition for all long-term workers since they usually offer better pay, fringe benefits, and controlled working conditions. It has been suggested by administrators that nursing homes tend to use younger workers, since their jobs often involve heavy lifting, whereas home care staffs tend to be older. But as institutions continue to discharge to the community or reject many chronically sick persons as bad insurance risks, the age differential may change (Banazak-Holl and Hines 1996).

Staff and Labor Force Issues

Turnover averages 10–12 percent a year but according to one study nearly a fifth of home-care agencies have rates above 25 percent and, according to other reports, the rate can rise to 60 percent for some agencies. The costs of turnover have been calculated to total $3,362.00 for each turnover (recruiting, screening, orientation, training, etc.). The major issues are recruitment of competent staff and reduction of the high turnover. Total labor costs, including benefits, are high in any labor-intensive service, despite low hourly wages.

The labor force of home care services present other difficulties. When workers are employed by an agency and placed in a patient's home, it is difficult to separate paid service from the traditional unpaid family care of the past. It has not clearly defined what kinds of special skill or training are needed beyond native human skills plus minimal information about a client, comparable to that required for employing a maid. Moreover, clients and their families generally do not place a high value on such staff. House cleaning experience, while not without skill, is not sufficient to care for a disabled or frail person living in his or her home. More is needed, for example, how to transfer a partly helpless individual, how to monitor medications. Relatives and neighbors can learn such additional skills, but it is more difficult to safeguard a partly dependent individual from physical abuse, theft, or neglect when the helper is a stranger. (See Chapter 3 for discussion of family roles.)

Who Are the Workers?

The most comprehensive study of home-care workers (Feldman 1988; AARP 1988) found that 95 percent are women working part time (an average of 29 hours a week). Half are drawn from minority populations, especially African American and Hispanic. Ethnicity varies by location and profession. For example, in rural areas the number of Caucasians who work as aides and kitchen help and as nurses may be high. Professional personnel have a different ethnic mix. But if we look only at home care, this means that physicians and nurses who visit occasionally as part of a plan differ in ethnicity from home care aides who spend all of their working time in a patient's home.

The home care staff overall can be characterized as poor, female, and minority. Their pay is low: 75 percent earn under $4.85 an hour. Their median personal income is $7,000 annually, and 65 percent of them are their family's primary wage earner. By contrast, aides and workers in nursing homes earn a median hourly wage of $5.29 an hour. Hospital aides, likely to be drawn from the same labor pool, earn $7.12 an hour on average (Crown, MacAdam, and Sadowsky 1991).

Half of home care employees work less than full time for any one agency and 20 percent work at more than one job. They lack health insurance or other benefits: only 19 percent have any health benefit from their job and 22 percent lack any form of health insurance. The compensation they receive is eroded by the fact that over half must use public transportation to go from client to client and are not paid for travel time. They may have several clients (2–3) a day. They are at risk of loss in work when a supervisor reports that a scheduled client for that day has been moved to a hospital and no replacement "case" is available, reducing the day's earnings by a third or more.

Home care workers are poorly educated. Forty percent completed eighth grade but 40 percent failed to complete high school. Their life responsibilities and conditions make it virtually impossible to take the time to complete their education or to acquire any other special skills no matter how much they might seek it (Feldman 1988). Three-fifths of home care workers are heads of households, in effect manning two households simultaneously.

The Personal Aides Work

The less skilled worker's tasks and working conditions are little understood and together they explain many of the manpower problems of turnover rates as high as 60 percent annually. The job is generally a lonely and often boring one. The worker is in another's home but not as that other's employee. The worker's job is not clearly defined and can range from cleaning up a house to cleaning up an incontinent person. The chronic sick and disabled are helpless in some aspects of daily life. They are often "unlovable" and difficult in behavior, but they are also in need of loving care. There is little preparation for either patient-client or worker in how to manage or handle the behavioral and less pleasant aspects of the job. The rapid turnover means that workers can change often for any one client. Training and supervision by the employing agency are skimpy. Training, which the employer must pay for, involves "down time," when the worker also loses pay because he or she is not seeing a client.

Members of the patient's family often misconstrue the job and treat the aide as a servant rather than as an employee doing a difficult job, which they, as family, do not want to perform but about which they may feel either guilty or uncomfortable. The work may be physically demanding, such as moving and transferring a client. Some studies suggest that health care of any kind is one of the more dangerous occupations as regards injury.

All this with inadequate pay. It is therefore surprising to find in the few serious studies of workers attitudes that many find real satisfactions in their jobs. Some feel that they are doing good in helping another in trouble, perhaps motivated by religious beliefs. Some develop an affectionate relationship with their client. Feldman's studies found that overall 84 percent were relatively satisfied. A majority found that supervisors and agencies treated them well although such ratings may reflect a reluctance to complain for fear of losing a job.

The major dissatisfactions were with low pay, lack of insurance benefits, and uncertain hours. Some are troubled by their isolation from other workers and from supervision. Many complaints could be reduced if pay were better and more stable and the tasks more varied (Feldman, 1988).

One of the unproved features of the field is the tendency to carve up tasks into separate compartments that may not make sense to anyone actually on the job. For example, an aide may be barred from moving a client, from doing minor house repairs, while a chore worker is limited to minor repairs or moving the furniture. Can an aide monitor a client's use of medication or take temperature?

The position of a personal aide is also confused by its relation to the number of other, more skilled specialists who may come and go at any time: a supervisor, a nurse to change a bandage or to check blood pressure, a home meal delivery, a chore worker to clean the walks, etc. Some of these are tasks that any family usually can perform for itself but in home care the emphasis is on varieties of protection. There is always the risk of fraud, abuse, and neglect but also the risk of too much complexity in work assignments, especially when the client isn't really in control of his or her household any longer.

Recruitment into the home-care labor force or the "secondary labor market" is marked by low wages, little chance of advancement, and little employment security—a labor market without much future but always needed. Although some surveys indicate that workers can find a good deal of satisfaction from intrinsic aspects of the job, the extrinsic aspects of the work are dominant. The workers remain poor, ill educated, doing work not much valued. Because long-term care for the disabled and short-term care for the ill have become a more significant part of both health and welfare systems, the time may be at hand to consider how the home-care dimension can be approached to minimize the weakness of its labor force.

Why Improve the Work Force and Conditions of Work?

As the needs of the disabled loom more important in community life, it would seem self-evident that a satisfactory system of care at home is in the interest of patients and their families and critical for the economic viability of provider agencies. This satisfactory system would rely heavily on labor-intensive inputs and on suitably trained and satisfied staff.

It is uniquely difficult to build such a home-care system because of several obstacles, some already alluded to. The border between family care and least-skilled maid service and a reliable personal care service is blurred. The field straddles both medical and welfare systems for financial support, but the public's regard for service and its willingness to pay treat the two differently. One is valued as being highly professional (medicine and nursing), and the role of the least skilled staff is not understood. Medical care is highly regarded and rewarded; welfare less so. And the two fields are burdened by numerous agencies and policies each addressing limited components of care and with inadequate mechanisms to link the parts smoothly together.

Despite all the obstacles, there have been continuous efforts to improve home-care manpower, which translates into improved home care for the emerging era when life at home for the disabled is a norm, not an aberration (U.S. Department of Labor 1990).

Demonstrations and New Proposals

The most common efforts are directed at improving pay and working conditions in order to increase recruitment, retain employees, and satisfy clients. Raising pay and benefits is limited by the marginal profitability of home-care agencies standing alone. Training workers results in lost work time, which reduces income and increases unit costs. Pay increases are limited by intense competition to attract patients where low cost is important, by what payers (both public and private) are willing to pay, and by what public payers demand to award contracts to the lowest bidder. Plans by major national chains of agencies to improve local management without raising pay or fees has sustained the serious weakness in local agency management because to do so would raise costs substantially (MacAdam 1993; Linsk, Kreigher, and Simon-Rusinowitz 1992).

Improvements in working conditions seem to have a slight effect though they are not sufficient to alter the industry patterns, given the force of economics in the secondary labor market. At least up to 1997 the disappearance of so many jobs at adequate wages (above poverty levels) for low-skilled workers created a large enough unemployed worker pool to limit efforts to raise wages. Competition from better-paying health institutions is also a factor.

Suggested Remedies

The costs of doing nothing about the labor force problems show up in high turnover, difficulty in recruiting, inadequate staffing levels, and recruiting only the least promising workers. Training is the universal panacea that has limits. At the aide level it can be demeaning and simplistic and can fail to produce self-worth about the job, or it can be the way to move rapidly up a career ladder, further increasing turnover. And it is costly in down time as well as instructors' salary.

The future of home service will ultimately depend on its labor force, capable and trusted by consumers sufficiently to assure a competitive edge among the alternatives for managing disability. Feldman's survey, reported in 1988, concluded with the following actions to improve the situation.

1. Employers should concentrate on recruiting more mature workers. Young workers are less satisfied with their jobs and able to move from job to job more readily than older ones.

2. Screening of new applicants should be done carefully. Most screening is rudimentary, based on few minutes talk or reliance on employed workers to bring in new candidates. If management has the skill, more sophisticated screening could give more attention to an applicant's willingness to work alone, to work with the disabled who present special behavior problems, and to forgo the value of being viewed as part of a team.

3. Programs that develop special skills in training and attention to creating career tracks in the system as training advances should be in place. Training in skills to handle "problem cases" may have special value for worker by giving them transferable skills but may also lead to more turnover unless career advances are possible.

4. Better supervisory help should be available for the worker who must handle substantive decisions about care made by professional workers who come periodically from other agencies—nurses, therapists, and the like. This involves professional staff learning to respect the functions of the aide, and the aide acquiring the self-respect about the nature of his or her place on a "team" even if that term is used very loosely. It is easy for a professional visiting briefly to give instructions to an aide, but when there are several different professionals, the aide may have to reconcile several conflicting directives. As in a patient's home, the care recipient may be the "boss" to whom the aide really listens, or the aide may misunderstand instructions not fully explained. So misunderstandings accumulate.

5. Minority workers who, for understandable reasons, may be especially sensitive to being assigned difficult cases, warrant special training and supervisory attention.

6. Pay differentials as rewards, expanded benefits, and tangible recognition of status by uniforms, and special awards make some difference, but work slowly and only for long-time workers. If a career plus pay and benefit increments are in place, it becomes more costly for the worker to leave but also more costly for the agency to keep the worker. The competitive and reimbursement environment makes a difference.

7. Full-time work, a salary in effect rather than an hourly wage, could change the episodic nature of the work force behavior. Those who work several jobs might be more stable if guaranteed full-time work and pay. Where an agency has many short-term and short-visit cases, a guaranteed pay may not be feasible.

8. Developing special workforce units may be possible in larger agencies. For example, a small cadre of full-time workers able to fill in on emergencies and difficult cases, receiving special pay and recognition, could be useful, but scheduling is extremely difficult.

9. Developing opportunities for career advancement makes demands on management but can have long-term advantages. A "clinical" track brings workers closer to paraprofessional tasks, which are more valued and respected and increase workers' pride. For the field, such career developments would be an asset. For the training agency it would require balancing compensation of some kind. A career in agency supervision is also a useful track, in effect an administrative in-service training track.

10. External political pressure from unions and others to raise pay may have an effect on the reimbursement and appropriation practices of payers and local governments.

11. Several public policy decisions would help. States could change nurse practice acts to permit aides to perform a wider range of services, with some training short of full nurse qualification.

12. States that permit clients to employ their own aides make training and labor force control difficult. A move to reimburse only through vendor agencies has been proposed, but some advocacy groups resist this as an invasion of a client's right to choose his or her own aide. Unions on the other hand may support such a move. Agencies may be wary of unions but they can be a helpful buffer between an agency and its publics. Aides are easily exploited and are especially vulnerable unless the low-skill labor supply is very tight. So reimbursement to the client/patient is good or risky depending on who is viewing the experience.

13. Contract bidding rules should be changed to exclude low bids based on substandard (by local standards) wages. Several ideas have been proposed but few have been systematically pursued.

14. New sources of workers may be found among younger retirees and mature workers who have lost jobs because of corporate restructuring. People who have retired but seek work have been considered. With industrial downsizing, especially for blue collar workers, this disemployed group might be a source, but the pay level and the lack of respect for home care work are all discouraging.

Licensing is a common method for raising quality standards and for protecting interests. To be effective, as, for example, in using training staff to raise standards of work and compensation, it is necessary that agencies be induced to adopt the standards in more than perfunctory ways. Is there inspection and how burdensome is it? Does better pay follow training mandates of licensing? If it does, it interferes with the labor market. If it does not, there is not much incentive for workers to take training before applying for a job or to take on-the-job training seriously. Licensing experience has shown that to work it has to be made to work.

A quite different solution has been tested in a very few cities—the launching of worker-owned and -managed cooperatives. At least one such agency in New York has been successful. It is difficult, however, to secure the capital to launch such a risky enterprise. Moreover, the worker-owners must understand the need to secure and work with excellent management if they lack those skills, as is likely and as demonstrated in other worker-owned companies.

Basic Restructuring of the Home Care "Industry"

Given all the complexities and obstacles, we have proposed experiments in a basic restructuring of the field moving from reliance on each provider agency to handle its own staffing to a community or regional agency to assume responsibility to develop a wide manpower approach; this can also move the field closer to parity with its more influential health field partners. Such a home care manpower agency could also develop career ladders on a regional basis and smooth out some of the difficulties in recruiting and retaining staff.

This approach builds on the past surveys and efforts to deal with manpower as reported by Feldman and others. It differs in the proposition that home care, by comparison with the health field, has remained a small agency field, undercapitalized, relying on a secondary labor force, without the means to influence either financing, training, promotion, or management, even when the service vendor is associated with a chain of vendors.

Priorities for Improving Labor Supply for Home Care

Feldman lists both general guides and specific steps for improving the workforce for home care. For concrete planning on labor, we suggest the following order of priorities:

1. Improved training for staff recruited

2. Interagency or regional cooperation to recruit and train staff and to develop incentives for retaining competent recruits

This may include experimentation with any or all of the following (lacking tested proof of efficacy of any one):

1. Individual incentives for better performance such as pay raises or promotion; higher wage rates at least to meet nursing home levels; experimentation with an annual wage rather than per hour/per case rate to minimize erratic earnings resulting from case cancellations, travel, and down time; significant recognition of value such as promotions and public recognition.

2. Organizational incentives: rationalize labor force use on a regional basis by regional agreements among home care agencies to reduce costs.

Chapter 12 outlines steps to meet the challenges that major restructuring in the health field has introduced, especially large combinations of services under one management or in one integrated system of multiple services all linked together systematically. Most of these services are medical and rehabilitative, with a short-term perspective using mostly skilled staffs, but they include nursing homes, which come closer to the home care mission, and some now include home care agencies for relatively short periods of posthospital care, all in the interests of containing costs and assuring continuity of service and management of a larger population base.

CHAPTER 5 ❋ *Cash versus Services:*
Putting More Home into Home Care

IN THIS CHAPTER we address a fundamental question: How best to organize and pay for home care services so that they optimize the control a handicapped client or patient has over his or her home environment. It is our view that control over the use of one's resources, or freedom of choice, is the desired norm and more closely approximates normal living conditions. Those handicapped persons who have adequate personal or family resources probably have the least difficulty in managing and supervising the home care services they require. Problems arise when an individual is clearly unable to manage the financial aspects, or when the family is negligent in fulfilling its responsibility. The issue is more serious for the population with limited resources. Therein lies a dilemma. If a community subsidizes an individual with public funds, how much or little control should it reasonably expect to exercise over how that public subsidy is used to realize its intended purpose? (Thurow 1974).

In this chapter, we concentrate on the population whose income is below the median national income of $35,000 a year. They are the most likely to need some subsidized help to pay for services at home. What follows explores the major variations in the demand for or potential use of home care and how the cash payment is both desirable and difficult to organize. We assume that most people prefer freedom in disposing of their income, whether their own or that acquired from a subsidized service for which they are eligible. But we also recognize that some individuals find so much autonomy difficult to handle either because of their disability or because of a history of dependency on others; at the same time payers, as trustees for the community, are skeptical and fear abuse of funds.

We also concentrate on provision of personal assistance services and related social supports. Personal assistants, their selection and pay are usually treated as measures of client/patient autonomy, which at the extreme translates into full control over choosing an aide, defining the tasks, changing aides, and paying as an employer. Even with adequate income, some clients can be either too ill or unwilling to act as employer and prefer to assign the task to someone else— sometimes a relative, more often a formal agency from which they seek the service and to which they can shift most responsibilities.

When medical and health services are also necessary, they are provided by a health care system in which it is accepted that major decisions are and should be controlled by professionals, although in recent years there has been an increase in patient participation.

Evolution and Extent of Public Cash Payments for Home Care

The use of a cash subsidy for home care is complicated because the home-care system uneasily spans two very different American human service systems— health care and welfare. The former is primarily concerned with treatment of acute illness, repair of injuries, prevention of disease and accidents, and promotion of good health. The complex medical judgments involved in these activities are traditionally the domain of skilled physicians or nursing professionals. Welfare, or income maintenance, has, in recent decades, been based largely on the social insurance model represented by Social Security, unemployment insurance, and workmen's compensation programs. After eligibility for a benefit or a service is established, the preferred financing mechanism has been a cash payment to the beneficiary. In the instance of public relief—those income maintenance programs designed to help the worthy poor who are unable to work—there remains a residue of the older tradition when the dependents were deemed incompetent to handle cash and received necessary help or services in kind. The historical arguments over cash versus services (or between indoor and outdoor relief) was only partially resolved in the matter of public relief; key decisions and management were provided by agency employees, even when financial help was given in cash or by voucher. This tradition has its roots in the view that dependent persons are so vulnerable that either they cannot perform normal home and selection tasks or the provision of a cash benefit is subject to abuse and likely to be used for purposes other than those intended.

Social or public provision to help the disabled live in their own homes with cash subsidies dates back at least 55 years in the United States, with enactment of the Veterans Administration Homebound and Attendance Programs authorized in November 1951 by Public Law 82-149.

A survey of Medicaid practices in providing home care in 50 states was conducted in 1984 and 1988 by the World Institute on Disability, including in-depth studies in six states. This has been supplemented by a 1993 survey of practices for the elderly in 3 states by the Commonwealth Fund (Doty, Kasper, and Litvak 1991; Litvak, Heumann, and Zukas 1987).

Beginning in 1970 the Levinson Policy Institute of Brandeis University initiated a ten-year exploration with demonstrations in several states and analyses of the subject concentrating first on the concept of home care as an efficient and cost effective alternative to the nursing home for long-term care through use of nonmedical social support services (Morris 1971; Caro 1973; Sager 1976). In the 1980s, a number of health policy analysts suggested that cash allowances could be a more appropriate and cost effective way to provide for the disabled needing long-term care (Brecher and Knickman 1985; Firman 1983; Grana 1983; Gruenberg and Pillemer 1981; Meltzer 1988; Scanlon 1992; Cameron and Firman 1995).

Beginning in 1979, several state governments initiated demonstration or statewide programs of diverse kinds to test the feasibility and utility of cash payments in some form: Colorado 1979, Wisconsin 1980, New Hampshire 1993 and Pennsylvania. In 1994, the National Council on Aging and the University of Maryland, with a grant from the Robert Wood Johnson Foundation began a study of the subject in both Europe and the United States. Recent European experiments and national policies date from at least 1980.

Summary of the Medicaid Approach to Client Autonomy

Despite its limitations, a cash approach has been influenced by the Social Security program for the permanently and totally disabled. It adds to the usual basic income security for food and shelter a subsidy to purchase necessary equipment and personal assistance services to make it more feasible for the long-term disabled to function in community life as do the able. And it proposes that the cash or subsidy be paid directly to the disabled individual. In cases of incompetence, a designated payee is provided for the client.

In the examples noted next, the purpose has been to combine more individual control, choice, and autonomy or responsibility with control over costs (data are largely based on the reports of the World Institute on Disability surveys of Litvak, Heumann, and Zukas 1987; Cameron and Firman 1995).

A major source of experience is the cluster of personal care service programs operated by state Medicaid agencies; these encourage experimentation with various arrangements, including cash payments in lieu of services delivered by an agency and use of various independent contractors or providers of personal assistance. State demonstrations were not always intended to enhance consumer control although that was one consequence. But political concern about increases in public spending and a desire to limit administrative and service costs have always been major limiting considerations. The number of persons covered by cash programs has tended to decline for all Medicaid personal care services.

Twelve programs used independent providers (i.e., not employees of a public agency), 10 of which permitted consumers to hire and fire their attendants. But only 3 allowed consumers to participate in paying the attendants. Personal attendant services can be arranged for in several ways. A public agency may employ, assign, supervise, and pay them. The state can pay a nonprofit or proprietary agency to perform these functions with contracted reimbursement. Or the agency can pay a relative or nominee of the client treating each one as an independent contractor, not an agency employee. Or cash can be provided to the client. The amount of client authority in any arrangement can vary. Personal care services are an option for both elderly and younger disabled eligible populations. In 1994, expenditures for personal care totaled $3 billion (Doty 1986).

Medicaid agencies can also secure other waivers to use Medicaid funds more flexibly to increase home- and community-based home care services primarily as a way to reduce public spending by opening up alternatives to nursing home admission as long as total expenditures do not rise. About two-thirds of these waiver funds go for the mentally retarded and developmentally disabled. Since these approaches are limited to those found eligible for a means-tested service, they are not an answer to home care for the larger population. The populations selected for personal care by any means are relatively small and popularly seen as "worthy needy." Overall, the encouragement to experiment is sharply limited by the key criterion that each option be budget neutral, placing the incentive on cost reduction.

This cash option, although attractive for many reasons, is not often used, as we will see. On the positive side, an individual is able to draw upon family and relatives to help and to compensate them for giving up their opportunities to work in the commercial world or working harder to look after both their patient and their other needs. They can also draw upon neighbors and friends. So administrative costs for supervision, recruiting and training staff, and maintaining records are reduced. By some estimates these savings to the payer agency can amount to about 30 percent (Doty 1986).

There is also a correlation between client control and the proportion of attendants who were previously known to or related to the client. In Michigan, 49 percent of the aides were relatives and 22 percent were friends of the client. Clients co-sign checks for their aides, who are treated as an employee of the client. This also permitted the state to avoid legal responsibility for withholding taxes. There is also some indication that client satisfaction with the service is higher in states that provide a greater measure of client participation in control (Doty 1986).

There is policy concern, and formal agency staff concern, that quality is less important in the client selection of aides than the political and fiscal conse-quences of abuse, fraud, and neglect via tort lawsuits. It is not clear that full con-trol of the home care function through licensing attendants or control through public employment of aides improves quality of care, at least when client satis-faction is factored into the criteria.

Surveys in 1988 and 1990 of 35 or more jurisdictions found that 70 percent of them permitted payments to family caregivers in varying ways (Linsk, Kreigher, and Simon-Rusinowitz 1992). Other states usually cited Health Care Finance Administration regulations. But an effort to prohibit a very wide range of rela-tives from being paid by Medicaid as caregivers was defeated in 1995, when the administration limited the restrictions states could impose on paying legally responsible relatives as caregivers.

Enhanced client control is still sharply limited by other federal and state reg-ulations. During the 1980s and early 1990s federal regulations governing Med-icaid required that personal care services programs be prescribed by a physician and supervised by a nurse. In 1993 the Omnibus Budget Reconciliation Act removed this requirement, which had been used to deny client selection and supervision of their personal attendants, although states were still empowered to require professional supervision if they wished. The issue is who decides who is a family caregiver. The Health Care Finance Administration first sought to define the term sharply but after 1995 decided to leave that decision up to each state.

On balance, the waivers have increased a home care constituency, but they directly affect relatively few beneficiaries. In 1987, 37 states had waivers, but they served only 59,000 elderly (Neuschler 1987). (See Chap. 10.)

Aides hired by clients receive slightly less hourly pay than do agency employ-ees. In 1988, personal attendants employed by a government agency averaged $8.00 an hour whereas independent providers earned an average of $4.59 an hour and employees of private agencies $6.02. For a systems' workforce, the im-plications are clear: will cash systems improve the conditions of the work force?

Some State Examples

Montana's Medicaid personal care services program began in 1977 using attendants employed by a county agency. In 1979, as caseloads grew, it began to permit clients to recruit their helpers and this became the dominant mode very
quickly. The state was relieved of the duty to pay taxes or be legally responsible
since the aides were "independent contractors." But after 9 years, the state required all aides to be employed by a certified agency. The reasons for the change
were the difficulty in overseeing the independent workers and their results; the
rapid rise in the caseload; and, legal rulings that the state remained responsible
for withholding taxes and other taxes for workmen's compensation and unemployment insurance, even though it had no way to monitor payments by the
client or aide. Within four years, the public funds paid to contract agencies for
employees rose from $3.85 an hour to $7.75, of which 30 percent went for administrative costs. Since the program was required to constrain overall Medicaid spending, the state began also to reduce the maximum number of attendant hours it would allow, from 70 to 40 hours a week (Doty 1986). The shift
was further encouraged when states found that they could be held legally liable
for actions of the client-hired independent aides. To protect against tort actions,
the state resumed more control.

Some states, such as Massachusetts, experimented with paying for personal
attendant service only when provided through a personal care agency, which
was required to have a governing board composed of at least 51 percent recipients, family members, and those with disabilities. These agencies took over administration of tax withholding, supervision, and the like. More states, such as
Texas and Maryland, opted to introduce a third party to manage care. Professional supervision was assured (1) by requiring that all employees be part of a
Medicare- or Medicaid-certified home health agency; and (2) by using state or
regional managers to determine eligibility or nurses to do assessments and to
monitor performance. In Maryland the nurse monitors also trained attendants
and checked on client complaints.

In 1993, New Hampshire began its small Self-Determination Project. It was
initiated in response to dissatisfaction of consumers, growing waiting lists for
home care, and the high costs of supporting the disabled by existing measures.
The project was phased in over three years to include a total of 45 clients, as
many as the state could plan on. The pool consisted mainly of the developmentally disabled of any age. The client has complete autonomy to decide how a
budget drawn from a state allocation will be used, but decides in consultation
with a personal agent and a circle of friends. Plans are subject to approval by the

state agency. Each case budget has a ceiling of 75 percent of what was previously paid on behalf of the client from state funds. The remaining 25 percent is reserved in a pool for emergencies.

The Colorado Home Care Allowance was introduced in 1979 as part of the old age pension program. It was created as an entitlement, but by 1988 the program had grown so large that the legislature set a limit on the funds available. A physician establishes the medical and functional condition for eligibility and financial eligibility is based on criteria for old age pension or aid to the needy blind or disabled. A caseworker decides if the patient is at too great a risk for self-management, whether existing informal care is sufficient and the frequency of visits. Relatives can be chosen by the client as an attendant. The program has an average per person monthly payment of $198.00 and is the least costly long-term care program in the state.

The Wisconsin Community Care Option dates from 1981. It is funded on an "as available" basis and covers all ages and all disabilities of persons eligible for or at risk of entering a nursing home within six months. Disability and eligibility are assessed by a nurse or a social work team, which spells out what is necessary for the client to remain in the community. The state concluded that a separate cash benefit is unnecessary since the budget agreed upon with each client gives the client choice in the attendant provider to be employed, as well as the services needed and their duration. Attendants or agencies that provide the services are paid by a check in the provider's name but sent to the client who uses it to pay out. The rates of pay range from $4.90 to $7.75 an hour. A county agency acts as fiscal agent so that the client can be treated as the employer for hiring, paying, and training but is relieved of the usual employer obligations in handling tax deductions and the like. The Wisconsin plan is basically a traditional welfare program but with great flexibility in budgeting the extra funds to incorporate special needs of the disabled living at home.

The Housebound Program and the Aid and Attendance Program of the U.S. Department of Veterans Affairs dates from 1951. It is a little recognized example of constructive pioneering by a federal agency. Veterans with a service-connected disability need only pass a disability test. Other veterans are means-tested. Spouses are also eligible. The eligible veterans are already in receipt of some benefit. The disability programs increase these benefits by $145.00 to $391.00 a month, depending on the basic pension program involved. An evaluation in 1983 found that the care received in the cash system was at least as secure as in the service in-kind system, which tends to counter the fear that the disabled will not use their added benefits for necessary care.

With all this history and the slow relaxation of constraints on efforts to widen cash payments to clients in order to increase their control over home care, it remains clear that there are difficult issues yet to be resolved. Not the least is the concern that state governments have that somehow home care will grow without control if clients have greater influence in picking and managing their own care paid from a public subsidy. Clients with their own resources are not so limited, but there is a long-standing history of skepticism about the amount of control to be given to those persons dependent on public help, either because they are not to be trusted or because public control over tax spending is eroded.

Numerous other arguments pro and con have been advanced and are still unresolved: public officials are concerned by scandals from even rare or scattered cases of abuse of tax funds by recipients; advocates worry that cash payments may be lower than a client's full needs, and some will suffer; others worry that cash payments may be subtly inflated out of reason by increasing the number of hours of service required by the moderately disabled. For labor, individual negotiations lose the advantages of group bargaining although there are costs to negotiating group rates.

Frequently, public uncertainty about cash payments leads to continual and unnecessary assessments of every case, raising the costs of a cash program unnecessarily.

Attendants, usually minorities and poor, may be vulnerable to irregular payment and loss of Social Security and other payroll withholdings, depriving the attendant of benefits.

Despite the gain in client satisfaction, when they do assume much of the management of their income and there is savings in public administrative costs, there remains the reality that not all handicapped persons seek this amount of freedom and may prefer to rely on someone else to take over the responsibilities when their health begins to sap their energies. A 1994 survey of 2,029 elderly in Massachusetts who were in some form of managed care or served fully by agency-provided services found that fully a fourth were not aware that they had or knew their case manager (Glickman, Stocker, and Caro 1997). Sixty percent acknowledged a need for a case manager to help them. But 33 percent reported they would be quite comfortable with less case management without objecting to it as a part of their service.

But, more important, about 20 percent showed active interest in assuming greater control in general. More narrowly, 39 percent would like, or not object to, scheduling their care plan; 24 percent might discharge their aide if necessary; and 18 percent would be more involved in determining the type and amount of services they received.

Such opinions need to be evaluated against the fact that the respondents who want more involvement were those in better health or were less satisfied with their services. There is room, therefore, either to try to improve the present professional direction or to test wider client autonomy whenever client satisfaction is the issue. The tangle of factors and interests lends itself to careful testing on a large scale. Complexity of issues need not preclude further search for effective solutions.

In the real world, the economics and accountability issues are equally or more decisive in choosing. If client autonomy, as measured by these examples, leads to escalating use and cost, what are the criteria to be for supporting the increase and the autonomy. But if those with their own resources control their affairs and prefer to, even when it increases the cost of home care overall by greater use and higher salaries, is it fair that only those with low income should be limited in their autonomy? One group may increase the gross domestic product and total spending, while the other affects the public budget. Policy choices are usually made on the basis of financial and political considerations, but in the background may lie ethical questions about fairness as well. At the height of the social insurance model, the aim was to have a program covering all, regardless of income. In the 1990s, with severe financial constraints and a large national deficit, the division of choice by class and income seems to widen.

More serious is the problem of accountability. Some policy makers fear that cash for home care may become an indirect way for relatives to begin drawing public benefits, or that traditional family responsibility to care for their own will be rapidly eroded and increase the amount of public dependency. There are also concerns that states will remain legally responsible for tax withholdings or for legal damages, even if the attendant is an employee of the client and not of the state.

So the movement to expand a cash system continues, but slowly. The apprehension may be encouraged by the 1960–80 English experiments in attendance allowances that became too costly for the public budget. But a 1990s demonstration and research effort conducted by the National Council on the Aging is trying to launch several state demonstrations based upon recent evidence from the United States and experience in several European countries. A parallel cash and counseling demonstration administered by the University of Maryland is funded by the Robert Wood Johnson Foundation and the federal government (U.S. Department of Health and Human Services 1990). The two initiatives are now coordinated.

Some European Experience—Types of Cash Program

When, as today, there is uncertainty about the direction for social policy, the experience of other industrialized countries that have evolved stable social programs or innovative new programs can at least stimulate fresh thinking (Cameron and Firman 1995).

DISABILITY ALLOWANCES OR CASH SUPPLEMENTS

Cash supplements to existing authorized grants compensate for the purchase of necessary services. These were usually offered first to war veterans. In 1974, 47 countries provided some form of "attendance allowance supplement" or "constant attendant allowance" under disability programs like the Old Age and Disability Insurance program. By 1981 there were such programs in 59 countries. If work injury programs are included, 95 countries have such arrangements (Grana 1983).

Eligibility requires loss of work and permanent incapacity requiring help with activities of daily living. Eligibility is usually determined by the patient's physician or other official. Payment levels vary by degree of functional disability, usually according to a national standard. They may vary with age or be based on a percent of a disability pension or a percent of previous earnings.

Because of fiscal constraints, England's early relatively generous cash attendance allowance system of the 1960s was later replaced by a national plan for a more flexible community-care program, which drew in part on the experience of the U.S. Channeling experiment.

CASH OR SERVICE OPTIONS

Examples of cash or service options are found in the German National Long-Term Care Program and two experiments in the Netherlands and Austria. In this model, clients are offered a choice between either services provided by professionals paid out of public funds and services delivered through a formal agency or a cash grant to use as they choose.

The Austrian Long-Term Care Allowance was enacted in 1992. It provides for cash payments ranging from $150.00 to $780.00 a month. It was introduced into a complex social insurance network in part to correct the balance between curative programs and long-term care programs. The former are well funded but terminate if no cure can be foreseen in the patient's case. The cash benefits depend on a physician's or other's assessment of need, and the sums paid do not reflect the cost of what is required. But individuals are generally free to use the benefit as they see fit. Almost all has been used to maintain existing informal caregiving arrangements. About 60 percent of the clients transferred the cash payment to their main informal helper, at least 30 percent of whom gave up their other work to devote themselves to the client. It did not lead to much increase in new caregivers.

The Netherlands has built on existing welfare relief systems in which the relief or pension budget authorized for a client who is found by professional tests to be functionally disabled can be augmented to allow for special needs as agreed upon with agency staff. Benefits in a client budget provided by a social welfare agency are increased to meet disability needs at home. A budget is negotiated with a case manager, the recipient, and his or her family and/or friends joining in the design of a care plan in which all share some role. The budget agreed upon is managed by the recipient and family or friends while the case manager regularly monitors the choices and results.

The German Long-Term Care Program is still evolving to help any disabled person secure permanent nonmedical assistance. The benefit is available from a home care agency. Cash supplements or payments range from $240.00 to $730.00 a month. The client can choose to receive the benefit through an agency; or directly. Caregivers can be recruited from among relatives or friends. In the cash option the payment is about half that given to an agency provider but sometimes the cash option exceeds the amount that would have been awarded to an agency. There have been reports that the government prefers the cash option as being less costly to the public sector. It is also a way for women with low earning potential to care for a relative at home instead of seeking paid employment. The devil is in the details.

Flexible Case-Managed Cash Benefit

A flexible model seeks to retain a firm organizational structure and control but does so by being flexible in how the budgeted sum is actually defined and used. It is mainly a case-managed program (with many variations) controlled by a staff worker but carried out through face-to-face discussions with each client to insure that client preferences are met within the funds allocated. Need is assessed professionally; the case manager links the client with support services provided by other agencies within their limitations and rules. Client advocates or friends join with providers on the client's behalf in defining what is needed and monitoring and evaluating the progress or its absence.

Private Insurance for Long-Term Care

Two major private insurers, UNUM and Aetna, began to experiment with coverage of long-term care in the 1980s by offering early versions of long-term care policies. By 1993, 135 third-party insurers have sold 2.3 million policies, and the number is still growing. The services covered are defined in each contract. Once disability and eligibility are determined, the insured can use benefits as he or she chooses. Some companies offer counseling separate from the persuasions of insurance sales staff, in order to help the client protect the benefits. There is usually periodic reassessment of a policy holder's condition. Policies may cover only home care or offer a choice between a nursing home and home care; the home care benefit is normally half the amount for an institution. Aetna originally offered a cash benefit as part of a group long-term care policy that permitted payment to an informal caregiver. UNUM, in one policy, paid for professional but not informal caregivers. (See Chapter 10 for additional discussion of private insurance for personal assistance.)

Private, for-profit insurance characterizes the recent movement in financing, either to complement or to replace the prior governmental efforts. It becomes a new version of public-private partnership on which so much of policy in America has been based. At the same time, momentum for a social insurance program for long-term care also developed. It finally failed as the conservative trend against enlarging government responsibilities came to dominate the political scene; however, at its 1980–94 peak, a large number of organizations joined a long-term care campaign, a high point of which was the introduction of the Pepper bill, a social insurance plan that would have added costs of between $10 and $50 billion dollars to public expenditure, depending on which populations would be covered.

Private insurance has built-in limitations. It appeals mainly to those financially able to pay the large premiums that most policies require because consumers are seldom ready to insure themselves against a contingency they will not confront until decades in the future. Private insurance also places first emphasis on medical treatments and prevention of disability. Most of the policies condition access to home care benefits on its link to active medical interventions. Although some also include by personal aides, home care is often framed as an alternative to nursing home admission. Since long-term care policies are sold competitively, they tend to avoid the very disabled or services not reimbursed by Medicare or Medicaid. Still the growth is sufficiently impressive to demand consideration for some populations at least. Beneficiaries are free to spend benefits as they see fit, once eligibility is determined by the insurer. Case management help is available, not mandatory. Some insurers offer expert counselling about the best way to use and conserve the benefits available. There is periodic reassessment of the beneficiary's condition and care. The policies may cover only home care, or they may offer options among nursing home, home care, and respite care. Many varieties are being market tested.

Aetna offered a cash benefit as part of its group long-term care policies. It also makes available a team of nurses and social workers to help a client plan the total program of care the company will cover; but the client remains free to choose. The home-care benefit is usually 50 percent of that paid for nursing home care. Payment to an informal caregiver is possible although usually the use of services from a licensed agency is required. In one of its policies, UNUM pays a percentage of the benefit for each day a professional home care service is used but not does not pay for informal caregivers. In a more comprehensive and costly policy, it pays for home care up to 50 percent of what it would pay for nursing home care (Aetna Life Insurance Co. and UNUM Life Insurance Co.).

Conclusions about Cash Benefits

At this writing, cash payment is an attractive option that satisfies many values, and it is supported by some evidence as to economy, reliability, and suitability. At the same time there are numerous cross currents of doubt not only among payers but also among beneficiaries. At best we conclude that there is more to be gained than lost in trying many more forms of cash payment in many more jurisdictions and for many more populations (Sabatino 1990). There will be at stake not only ideological beliefs about costs and preferences but also uncertainties about how far it is possible for home care to grow in competition with other programs also addressing long-term disabilities. More important, the outcome of a cash program may have much to do with public and private convictions about the value of life as near to normal as possible for the long-term handicapped of any age and the role they play in their own care. Except for Social Security, which is also being reassessed, private income sources characterize Americans' preference for personal control over income.

There is a practical labor issue to consider. It is reported anecdotally that clients who recruit and pay their own aides pay less than formal agencies do. In good economic times, finding personal assistance staff independently may be difficult.

CHAPTER 6 ✳ *Assistive Devices*

$\mathcal{I}$N THIS CHAPTER we will focus on the manner in which various assistive devices can extend the effectiveness of long-term personal-care services. Our perspective is that, for persons with disabilities, mechanical, electrical, and electronic devices and enhancements can significantly complement strategies that involve self-care or the assistance of others (Agree 1994). Assistive technologies can, for example, make a disabled person more self-sufficient in performing tasks of daily living, reduce the effort required of paid and informal caregivers, or enable caregivers to assist more efficiently. Assistive technologies can make living environments more suitable for people with disabilities, reduce threats to their safety, and make it easier to obtain assistance in case of an emergency.

The role of assistive devices in home care for the elderly has received relatively little research or policy attention. Informal caregiving, formal home-care services, and residential long-term care strategies have all received much more attention. Fortunately, the literature is well enough developed to be suggestive of the potential contributions of assistive devices and of the barriers to their more widespread use. In this chapter we will describe a variety of assistive technologies that are currently available as well as some of the problems associated with the development, production, and costs of assistive devices. Special attention is given to personal response systems because of the relatively well developed research literature on them. Personal response systems are both interesting in their own right and illustrative of challenges associated with other assistive devices. We conclude with a discussion about prospects for the future development of assistive devices.

Assistive technologies range enormously in their sophistication and cost. Some are bulky; others are tiny. Some require installation; others are freestanding. A wide range of tools can be classified as assistive devices. Devices that can be used to assist with mobility, for example, range from simple walking sticks to motorized wheelchairs with elaborate electronic controls. Some devices that are important resources for people with disabilities are also valuable aids for people without disabling conditions. Among these generally useful devices are elevators, electronically controlled door openers, and microwave ovens (Enders 1986; Bader 1994).

For much assistive technology, the physical device is only a portion of the technology. For personal response systems, for example, radio and telephone systems are linked to specialized communication and service systems. These systems are effective only to the extent that they have personnel available to receive emergency calls, to determine the nature of the emergency, and to deploy someone to follow up. Medication organizers are helpful only to the extent that they are regularly and carefully filled and conscientiously used. Computer-assisted shopping services require someone to assemble and deliver the goods that are ordered.

Even seemingly freestanding assistive devices may require considerable service support. If they are to be fully useful, glasses should have an accurate correction and a careful fitting. Glasses need replacement periodically to reflect changes in vision. Similarly, hearing devices need continuing battery replacements, regular cleaning, and periodic checkups. They are readily damaged if dropped. Regular hearing checkups are needed to assure that devices are properly calibrated. Battery-powered wheelchairs provide an example of a device that requires both training for use and continuing maintenance. Users must remember to recharge their batteries regularly. While batteries can be recharged easily by plugging recharging equipment into a wall outlet, users can also easily forget occasionally to do so. The resulting temporary loss of ability to use the equipment may be very frustrating.

Technological Aids and Their Uses

Our definition of assistive technology encompasses both physical objects and the purposes for which they are used. Some technologies are best conceived as means for coping with or overcoming the consequences of an impairment such as loss of vision, hearing, memory, and mobility. Glasses and contact lenses, for example, are widely used to compensate for loss of visual acuity. Hearing aids are conventional devices used by those who have experienced some hearing loss. An assistive device that provides visual cues, for example, color coding, may be used by those who have experienced memory loss. Those whose ability to walk has been reduced by weakness in the legs or loss of balance may be able to cope by using a cane, a walker, or a wheelchair.

Assistive devices may be simple or complex. It is useful to classify them according to the daily living tasks that they support. For example, aids available for those with difficulty in bathing include grab bars in tubs, wheelchairs designed for showers, and lifts that can be used to hoist a person with a disability into or out of a bathtub. To assist those with difficulties in toileting there are on the market disposable undergarments and elevated toilet seats. Devices used to help those with difficulty in dressing include clothing with easy-to-manipulate fasteners such as Velcro and extra-long shoe horns. For persons who have difficulty eating independently, there are easy-to-grip eating tools and no-spill beverage containers. For individuals with difficulty in transferring, there are both lifts and hoists and chairs that double as informal daybeds.

Kitchen tools are available to facilitate various tasks such as opening cans and bottles. Heating of food can be simplified greatly through the use of microwave ovens. For those with difficulty in taking medications as prescribed, containers have been developed in which medications can be organized by the day of the week and the time of day at which they should be administered. Electronic timers are also available that provide a reminder when medications should be taken.

For persons who experience difficulties in using the telephone, a wide range of assistive resources are available. Large print numbers on the dial or button pad make it easier for the visually impaired to dial a telephone. For those with memory difficulties, programmed dialing features may be helpful. For those with difficulty hearing the telephone ring, amplified ringing and flashing lights are available. Extra amplifiers are available for those with difficulty hearing the normal volume of telephone messages. For those with difficulty in handling the telephone, speaker phones and cordless phones are readily available.

Some assistive devices are most readily conceived as strategies for modifying a household environment to accommodate a person with disabilities (Salmen 1994). The construction of ramps and elevators, for example, can enable a person with disabilities to overcome obstacles to mobility in a household environment. Adaptive door handles may make it easier for those with difficulty in grasping and turning standard door knobs to move from one room to another. Enhanced lighting and hand railings may be important aids to prevent falls.

Personal safety is another useful focus for assistive devices. Personal response systems have been developed to enable the elderly and persons with disabilities who live alone to signal for help in case of an emergency. People with Alzheimer's disease who are at risk of wandering can be located more readily if they wear special tiny portable radio transmitters.

Product Development and Distribution

Because assistive technology has received very little comprehensive research attention in the home- and community-based long-term care literature, much of our discussion is inevitably impressionistic and speculative. To the extent that assistive technology has received attention, the focus has tended to be upon relatively specific needs and technologies (Agree 1994; Batavia and DeJong 1990). Jon Pynoos, at the Andrus Center at the University of Southern California, for example, has focused on shelter modifications. The Lighthouse in New York City has concentrated on aids for the visually impaired. Dibner (1992) has stimulated the development of personal response systems.

An impression that appears to be widely held among those who have focused upon this field is that the development of assistive strategies has greatly outpaced utilization (Bowe 1989). The general perception is that consumers are relatively unaware of the range of devices available and often do not make effective use of the devices that they possess.

Assistive devices are developed and distributed primarily through private markets. Effective distribution of specialized products to widely dispersed populations of disabled people is inherently challenging. Distributors use a variety of strategies. Some devices that assist with mobility are sold on a retail basis in stores that specialize in wheelchairs, crutches, and braces. These stores, however, do not characteristically sell a full range of assistive devices. Some are advertised in publications that reach older people generally. American Association of Retired Persons (AARP) publications, for example, regularly include advertising for some assistive products. Some distributors rely heavily upon professional gatekeepers. Occupational therapists, for example, are often in a position to make recommendations about mobility aids to older people who are recovering from fractures or strokes. It is in the interest of suppliers to keep occupational therapists aware of their line of mobility aids. Although audiologists usually do not sell hearing devices, they are in a position to recommend types of hearing devices and suppliers. Suppliers have reason to keep audiologists well informed about their products.

Distributors of assistive devices may not always find professionals fully helpful. Some professionals concentrate on a limited range of strategies. Opthalmologists and optometrists, for example, tend to concentrate on strategies that lead to better glasses or contact lenses for those with vision problems. They are likely to be helpful to distributors of better lenses. But they may not take initiative in informing patients about better reading lamps or sources of large-print publications.

An explicit link to health care is a critical element in the distribution of some assistive devices. When the use of specific devices is prescribed as part of a therapeutic regimen, its cost can sometimes be charged to Medicare, Medicaid, or a private insurer. For patients recovering from hip fractures, for example, the cost of a walker may be covered by insurance. When devices can be justified as necessary to support employment, state vocational rehabilitation funding may be available. For manufacturers and distributors of assistive devices, third-party coverage can be a major boost to distribution. The cost of most assistive devices, however, is not covered by a third party.

Another important distribution strategy for suppliers is to seek broader markets for assistive devices. Telephones with oversized key pads, for example, are successfully sold by general telephone retailers to people without severe visual impairments. Books on tape are another example of a product that in this instance was introduced for the hearing impaired but is now enjoyed much more widely. Medication organizers were developed for older people with multiple prescriptions and some memory difficulties. These simple devices, which are sold over the counter in most pharmacies, are useful for anyone taking a number of pills on a regular basis. Electronic reminders, nonskid surfaces for stairs, and kitchen gadgets for opening jars are other examples of products designed initially for people with disabilities that have been distributed successfully on a wider basis.

Distribution of assistive devices through broader outlets has major implications for price. If items can be marketed successfully to general populations, they can be sold at substantially lower prices than if they are distributed solely through channels that reach only the disabled.

Devices that are particularly helpful to people with disabilities but are primarily marketed to general populations pose other distribution issues. Examples include microwave ovens, beverage containers with nonspill lids, and pump dispensers for liquid soap. In these cases, the important question is how people with disabilities learn that the product is likely to be particularly useful to them. For the distributors of these products, the disabled may represent such a small, hard-to-reach population that special marketing efforts are not considered productive. In these instances, consumers may have to discover the products themselves or learn about them through professionals such as occupational therapists, mass media consumer advisors, or informal word of mouth.

An irony in the distribution systems for assistive devices is that price may have important implications for availability. More elaborate devices, which can command a higher price, may be more aggressively marketed than equally useful but much simpler devices. Without adequate profit potential, the simpler device will not be manufactured and distributed.

Consumer Access

Limited use of assistive technology can also be analyzed from a consumer per-spective. Andersen's model of health service utilization can be adapted to exam-ine the circumstances in which consumers use adaptive equipment (Andersen 1995). Following the Andersen model, several sets of personal characteristics of consumers can affect use of assistive devices. Receptivity is a highly pertinent dimension. The personal response system literature, for example, shows that denial of need is a major barrier to the introduction of assistive devices for older people residing in the community (Montgomery 1992). Family members and involved professionals may be convinced that assistance is needed, whether it is a service or a device, but be told firmly by the older person that no help is required.

The differences in availability of third-party financing also contribute to greater or lesser use of assistive devices on the part of younger populations. The vocational rehabilitation and educational funding for assistive devices that are available to younger populations are not available to older people with disabil-ities. Particularly among the elderly, individual capacity to make effective use of assistive devices can affect their use. Factors such as good general health, men-tal alertness, and high levels of motivation that are critical ingredients in suc-cessful use of technology by younger individuals with disabilities are less likely to be present among older people who develop disabilities gradually over time. Tendencies toward confusion and depression that are relatively prevalent among the elderly are obstacles to the effective introduction of assistive devices. All of these factors may contribute to the lower rates of use among the elderly with disabilities than among younger people with disabilities (LaPlante 1991).

Knowledge of the manner in which assistive devices can be used effectively is another potentially important barrier (Seeleman 1993; National Council on Disability 1993). Both the complexity of the problem and access to information about devices come into play here. From a consumer's perspective, specific self-care limitations may be addressed in a variety of ways. Useful for illustrative purposes is the situation of an older person living alone who has substantial difficulty in lifting and manipulating objects, in part, because of severe arthri-tis. This individual experiences difficulty in preparing meals. In the abstract, a variety of strategies may be useful including kitchen redesign to make a more efficient work environment, introduction of special tools such as an electric can opener, kitchen tools with easy-grip handles, and a microwave oven to facilitate cooking and heating food. A strategy that focuses only on food preparation is incomplete if it does not also address kitchen cleanup. In the situation described, simplification in food preparation may be at least as practical a solution as one that eases food preparation. Extensive reliance on prepared foods that require only heating may be a sensible strategy. Use of prepared foods and disposable plates and flatware may minimize the need for kitchen cleanup. In fact, the use of a home-delivered meal service may greatly reduce the need for both shopping and meal preparation.

A major question for consumers is the manner in which they identify and assess options for solving problems like the one described here. The premise is that individuals with disabilities can ordinarily work out their own solutions to challenges arising from self-care limitations. In other words with advice from family and friends, the older person is usually expected to be able to identify devices that promise to facilitate meal preparation, identify easy-to-prepare food, and services that deliver prepared food. On matters such as meal preparation, consumers ordinarily are expected to be able to learn about options by visiting retail stores, examining catalogs, and considering the advice available through the mass media. In this respect, consumers with disabilities are similar to other consumers. They should be able to learn about microwave ovens and electric can openers by visiting appliance stores. The involvement of professionals in assisting consumers with disabilities in developing strategies for coping with disabilities is by no means routine. Of interest are the circumstances in which consumers draw upon occupational therapists for advice about use of assistive devices or architects for advice about household modifications. Older people who are hospitalized because of traumatic incidents such as strokes or hip fractures are likely to receive rehabilitation services that include occupational therapy. When the onset of disability is gradual as tends to be the case with arthritis, consumer contact with professionals with expertise in assistive technology is much less certain. Relatively little is known about the quality of the solutions that consumers and their families are able to work out for themselves, the circumstances in which professional advice is sought, the extent to which professional advice is accepted, and the degree to which professional advice leads to improved solutions to daily living problems.

Cost can be an important barrier to the introduction of assistive devices. The cost of assistive devices varies enormously. The remodeling of kitchens and bathrooms to accommodate a person with disabilities may cost thousands of dollars. On the other hand some useful devices can be purchased at a very low cost. A tool to facilitate the opening of bottles and jars, for example, can be purchased for a few dollars. A telephone with an oversized key pad can be purchased for less than $50. Floor lamps with halogen bulbs that provide highly effective indirect room lighting can be purchased for under $30.

As indicated above, insurance sometimes eliminates or reduces cost as a barrier to the introduction of an assistive device. But insurance tends to cover the cost of assistive devices only when the devices are directly supportive of medical care. The cost of most assistive devices is not covered by medical insurance. In some instances, insurance covers the cost of a medical gatekeeper who can help to gain access to assistive devices. Health insurance, for example, may cover the cost of a visit to an opthalmologist who prescribes glasses, but the insurance is not likely to cover the cost of the glasses. Similarly health insurance may cover the cost of an audiologist's diagnostic services that yield a prescription for a hearing aid but not the cost of the device itself.

Some assistive devices are available to consumers without charge. In many communities, voluntary organizations serving specific disability groups such as the blind and the hearing impaired make certain devices available on a subsidized basis. On a highly selected basis, the federal government subsidizes some devices. Books for the Blind, for example, is a service offered by the federal government to all with visual impairments regardless of income. The service lends tape players, head sets, and audio tapes that are mailed to consumers and may be returned without charge.

When assistive devices are effective substitutes for formal services, they can sometimes justify relatively high cash outlays. If an older person uses ten hours a week of personal assistance services at $10 per hour, the cost on an annual basis would be $5,200. If an expenditure of $2,000 on various assistive devices to facilitate meal preparation and other household tasks reduced the need for personal assistance to five hours per week, the assistive devices would pay for themselves in less than a year. (The strategy would reduce annual expenditures for personal assistance to $2,600 resulting in a savings of $600 in the first year.)

Some consumers, of course, lack the financial resources to invest as much as $2,000 in adaptive devices. Uncertainties about time horizons can also discourage both consumers and third parties from investing in adaptive equipment. If, for example, the hypothetical older person required admission to a nursing home within three months, the equipment would not pay for itself. On the other hand, nursing home care is likely to cost over $3,000 per month. The high cost of nursing home care encourages even a risky investment that extends the viability of in-home care arrangements.

Installation and assembly are issues with some assistive devices. Hand railings and grab bars, for example, must be attached to walls. Because proper installation requires that they be firmly anchored, more is involved than superficially screwing them into walls. For the installation of some of these devices, a carpenter or skilled handyman may be needed. The inexpensive floor lamps that are available require assembly. Most adults are likely to be able to follow the directions in screwing the sections together, but a functionally disabled older person with impaired vision is likely to be dependent on someone else to assemble the lamp. Memory features on telephones may be useful for somewhat confused older people, but they are likely to need assistance from someone else in putting frequently called numbers in memory. They are also likely to need easy-to-follow instructions for their use.

Training and practice are often needed if assistive devices are to be put to good use (National Council on Disability 1993). Some instruction in the use of a device as simple as a walker, for example, is advisable. Fully alert adults and children can quickly learn to use a microwave oven. An older person with less familiarity with electronic controls may not be able to see or follow written instructions; instead some patient training over several days may be needed. Skill in cooking with a microwave oven is another matter. Successful cooking procedures for conventional stoves and ovens do not apply to microwave cooking. Adults typically can follow the literature that comes with microwave ovens to learn basic cooking procedures. They also often add to their skills quickly through trial and error. The capacity for self-instruction, however, cannot always be assumed. Some people with disabilities may not be able to learn from the written instructions and they may not be able to learn quickly enough through trial and error. Rather they are likely to require patient human training if they are to learn the basics of food preparation with a microwave oven. The source of the needed training is particularly uncertain when they live in relative isolation.

The need for training applies particularly to computers, which hold great promise for facilitating communication for people with disabilities. Even if some communication applications for people with disabilities are designed for easy use, some basic skills are necessary simply in turning the unit on, using the key board, gaining access to specific software, and turning the unit off. For many adults who did not grow up with personal computers, even the most basic use of computers continues to be intimidating. For older adults, training in the use of computers is a good deal more plausible strategy prior to the onset of serious disabling conditions than it is later. Realistically, the use of computers to aid the elderly disabled is far more likely for future generations of older people than it is for older disabled people today.

To the extent that resistance to adaptive equipment stems from a lack of confidence in one's ability to learn and general discouragement, training may be most effective if it is combined with strategies designed to build confidence.

Carefully orchestrated success experiences in using adaptive equipment can be used to build the confidence that leads to further efforts to master the use of the equipment.

A subtle but potentially important issue in effective use of adaptive equipment is personal or household organization. This applies, for example, to devices that are not in constant use. Consumers must be able to locate them when they are needed. In fact, reminders to use them can be helpful. Household organization is important even for those without disabilities. Unless the household is well organized, specialized kitchen tools, for example, may not be found when they are needed. Consumers may even forget that they have certain gadgets or do not think to use them for all the applications for which they promise to be helpful. The challenge of household organization escalates for those with limitations in vision, memory, and mobility. They are challenged to remember all of the devices that they have at hand, are more likely than others to misplace what they have, and find it more difficult to search for devices that are not readily found.

A key factor in successful use of adaptive equipment, then, may be very careful household organization to assure that needed devices can be found and that simple instructions for their use are also readily at hand. This implies that the living environment of some persons with disabilities requires more careful organization than conventional households. For many of those who become disabled in later life this implies substantial household simplification. Some people who have spent a lifetime acquiring possessions may have to eliminate some of them or store them away carefully so that the devices that are essential to day-to-day problem solving can be readily found. Reorganization may also be required to make needed devices readily available. Shelving, for example, may need to be lowered so that necessary equipment and supplies can be reached.

From a consumer's perspective, the effective use of adaptive equipment is likely to depend upon a combination of personal and structural factors. Such personal characteristics as alertness, energy, and motivation are likely to affect both receptivity to and success in use of devices. Structural characteristics including cost, availability of devices, ease of use, and household organization are also likely to affect use.

Interface with Human Assistance

In general, assistive devices should be seen as complementing rather than substituting for human assistance. The point can be illustrated with the meal preparation example used above. In principle, a person with disabilities can approximate self-sufficiency through the use of a shopping service to purchase house-hold goods, can prepare food independently in a kitchen especially designed with supplies and utensils readily at hand and equipped with a microwave oven, and can minimize cleanup by using disposable dishes. In reality, particularly with older disabled people, assistive technology is likely to be used in conjunc-tion with human assistance. In large measure, a shopping service involves hu-man assistance. A good deal of the food delivered by the shopping service is likely to be prepared food. In this case the human assistance is simply not visible to the consumer. Some meals may be home delivered whether ordered through a subsidized meal service or through a restaurant. Again human assistance is in-volved in meal preparation, but it is not visible to the consumer. The older con-sumer may do some kitchen cleanup after meals but rely upon paid help for more thorough kitchen cleaning. Human assistance is likely to be needed in removing trash. Use of prepared foods and disposable dishes, in fact, may in-crease the amount of trash that needs to be removed. Further, the older con-sumer may also greatly value the contact with the people who take shopping orders over the telephone, deliver household supplies, deliver hot meals, clean the living unit, and come occasionally to repair devices when they fail.

Because of effective use of assistive devices, a disabled older person may not need assistance daily in the household in meal preparation or for that matter with any other task. The larger picture, however, is that assistive devices shift the human assistance; they permit more efficient human assistance (food for many people, for example, can be partially or fully prepared in a single kitchen), move much of the assistance out of the household, and redistribute the timing of the assistance—to the convenience of the provider. For the consumer, the cost is lower than it would be if the food were prepared by paid personnel in the household.

The out-of-home food preparation solution has indirect consequences for consumers. When compared to in-home food preparation by a paid person, the consumer enjoys greater privacy but has less social contact when a food-deliv-ery person replaces someone who prepares a meal in the home. The implica-tions for consumer choice are uncertain.

Personal Response Systems

Because they represent a relatively new and distinct strategy that has received some analytic attention, personal response systems are useful in illustrating the potential of assistive devices. Personal response systems were introduced in 1973 in the United States by Andrew Dibner to enhance the personal security of vulnerable people living alone (Montgomery 1992). At the heart of the system is a tiny radio transmitter attached to an individual who can call for emergency assistance by pressing a button. The signals are monitored continually at a central location and help is dispatched rapidly when needed. Personal response systems have been introduced as an improvement over conventional telephone systems. The prototypical incident for which the system was designed is a fall. The system allows the victim to signal for help even when it is not feasible to get to a telephone. Further, the system sends a signal immediately to monitors whose sole concern is emergency assistance to the frail elderly and those with disabilities. Emergency telephone services, which are reached by dialing 911, in contrast, involve much more varied appeals for assistance. Personal response system monitors typically make an initial call to designated family members or neighbors who are asked to investigate. When necessary, emergency medical services are sent to the scene.

Personal response systems have been developed through private industry. In the United States, Dibner organized a firm, Lifeline, that developed the technology and distributed it. Subsequently, a number of competitors have entered the field. In the United States, hospitals have played a major role in the distribution by developing their own personal response systems. Hospitals are interested in sponsoring personal response systems as a way of maintaining a loyal patient base among the chronically ill elderly. In an article on personal response systems in the United States, a Lifeline executive explicitly illustrates the potential of personal response systems in generating revenue for sponsoring hospitals (Montgomery 1992).

Most fundamental, personal response systems are sold as a means of assuring that older people are safe living alone. They provide older people and their adult children with peace of mind that pleas for emergency help will be heard. Inquiries for alarm systems tend to be triggered by a negative event such as an accident or the death of a spouse (Breen 1992). Adult children often provide the impetus for introducing the systems.

Research conducted by Sylvia Sherwood and John Morris and summarized by Montgomery (1992) indicates that calls for assistance are relatively infrequent, averaging one in two years. The formal experiment conducted by Sherwood and Morris (1980) showed that among the severely functionally disabled elderly, the presence of the devices was effective in preventing nursing home placement. Further the costs of the personal response systems were more than offset by reduced costs of formal services (Ruchlin and Morris 1981).

By 1989, personal response systems were serving approximately 350,000 people in the United States at any one time. Duration of service was surprisingly short—approximately 10.5 months (Montgomery 1992). Clients terminate typically because they die or because they move to a nursing home. In 1990, equipment costs in the United States ranged from $500 to $800. Installation and training charges were from $30 to $175. Monitoring charges cost from $20 to $45 per month.

Personal response systems have achieved some success in establishing public third-party payment. In 1992, nineteen states included coverage of personal response services in their Medicaid home- and community-based services program (Montgomery 1992). New York State was planning to cover personal response services in its Medicaid-financed personal-care program (Montgomery 1992). The New York State personal-care program is a particularly notable application of personal response systems because until recently the New York program was extraordinarily generous in its service authorizations. In New York City in the 1980s, service authorizations for the home attendant program averaged approximately 50 hours per week (Caro and Blank 1988). Presumably, attendants were spending much of their time doing passive surveillance. If the personal response system in New York includes sound arrangements for following through on calls for help, the state is in a position to show that personal response systems can provide effective monitoring at a cost much lower than that provided by intensive attendant services.

A report on the New York City experience in using personal response systems as a basis for deep reductions in home care authorizations, however, indicates that the systems were not a fully satisfactory substitute for personal assistance services. As a result of a class action lawsuit filed on behalf of the Medicaid Home Attendant Program clients, New York City agreed to review its policy of limiting most clients to four hours of service a day and providing personal response system services. Advocates argued that the personal response systems were given to clients suffering from Alzheimer's disease and other debilitating illnesses who were incapable of using them. A lawyer for the plaintiffs was quoted: "Many of the tasks performed by a home attendant simply cannot be replaced by a personal alarm. Technology does not take you to the bathroom, help feed you dinner or help you get out of bed." The city agreed to give the personal response systems only to those capable of using them. Complaints about the city's deep reduction in maximum home care authorizations were not resolved, however (*New York Times*, April 18, 1996).

Significant technical advances have been made in personal response systems since their introduction (Dibner 1992). Voice systems with two-way communication have replaced nonvoice systems. The transmitters worn by users are now much smaller than they were originally. Personal response systems now have the capacity to do environmental monitoring, that is, they can detect smoke and temperature extremes. Further, they can be organized so that an alarm is triggered by lack of movement in a dwelling unit. Monitoring units now routinely use personal computers to maintain basic data about clients.

Personal response systems also illustrate the link between assistive devices and human assistance. The systems involve both radio transmitters and a monitoring service. When clients seek help, the service is only as effective as the monitors are successful in contacting family, neighbors, or volunteers to make initial inquiries and then seek medical backup when it is needed. In fact, the organization of an effective system for following up on calls for help may be more challenging than deployment and maintenance of the radio transmitters.

Personal response systems also invite further research on cost effectiveness. The experiment conducted by Sherwood and Morris (1980) may only show that personal response systems prevent or delay institutionalization because they provide older people, their families, and professionals with greater confidence in their safety. The degree to which they objectively improve safety is another matter. To what extent do customers report emergencies that they could not have reported by telephone? To what extent do personal response systems trigger emergency services that are quicker and more effective than community emergency services that can be reached by dialing 911? These are empirical questions that invite investigation.

Future Developments

Efforts to expand the use of assistive devices can take a number of directions including product development, distribution systems, and consumer access. If developments in the recent past provide a basis for future projections, we can anticipate some further gains in technology to assist the disabled. Where these gains will come is by no means clear.

Improved awareness of assistive devices among self-directed, self-financed consumers will lead to improved distribution. A number of national distributors publish illustrated catalogs with a wide range of moderately priced devices. Basic public education, which will lead to increased consumer awareness of these catalogs, is likely to stimulate increased use.

Efforts to use computers more extensively to improve communication are certain. We can anticipate, for example, that information about assistive devices and a wide range of shopping services will be available through computer networks. More complete product information should be available through Internet resources than through printed catalogs. In principle, opportunities for shopping via the computer should be particularly valuable for those with mobility limitations. Improved technologies for operating computers with voice commands may make computers more accessible to those who have difficulty in operating a keyboard or using a mouse. People with disabilities will be able to share their insights about adaptive equipment over the Internet. How widely consumers with disabilities will be reached by the Internet is uncertain. The extent to which the information disseminated via the Internet will prove to be useful is also not known. The cost of computers, the extent to which mature adults acquires skills in use of computers and the Internet, the cost of access to Internet services, and the cost of goods that can be purchased via the Internet will certainly affect access. Unless computer access is subsidized, many of the disabled are not likely to participate in the gains that can be expected through advances in computers.

Centers that maintain data bases on assistive devices and make information available to consumers on a drop-in or telephone basis, such as the Massachusetts Assistive Technology Partnership Center in Boston, warrant consideration. It maintains a great deal of information on strategies to assist the disabled. Some of the information is computerized; other information is organized in more conventional ways. An advantage of such a center is that its staff can provide answers to questions and advice that a consumer might not be able to find in searching a catalog or directory.

Distribution systems will remain important in extending the availability of assistive devices. For more complex devices, the key to effective distribution will remain the discovery of larger markets that make it possible to achieve dramatic reductions in unit costs and production. For this reason, the greatest potential lies in devices that are useful to people who are not disabled. For less complex devices, the challenge will remain finding a sufficient market and pricing so that there is incentive for devices to be supplied widely through private markets. Subsidized consumer education services may be needed on a continuing basis to assist the disabled in learning about low-cost technologies that are not effectively distributed through private markets or that are readily available, such as liquid soaps and pump dispensers.

Lowering the barriers experienced by individual consumers to the use of assistive devices will remain important. Efforts to extend consumer receptivity to assistive devices, to increase consumer knowledge, to improve consumer training in their use, to promote better household organization that is conducive to effective use of technology are all important directions for developmental efforts. Some gains in these areas are possible through general consumer education. Some are also possible through individual counseling of consumers.

Broadening the sensitivity of case managers who work with home- and community-based long-term care services for the elderly to include attention to assistive devices may be productive. Traditionally, case managers have been encouraged to concentrate on service strategies. In assessing home-care clients, case managers might be attentive, for example, to the need for devices that may be appropriate in light of impairments and daily living deficits. When devices need professional prescriptions, case managers might make appropriate referrals. For various deficits, however, case managers might be able to provide information about the range of products available and sources of products. When clients acquire assistive devices, case managers might help them with simple assembly and installation and provide them with training and encouragement in their use.

Case managers in home-care programs for the elderly can play a stronger role in encouraging the use of assistive devices. The Gerontology Institute at the University of Massachusetts in Boston in collaboration with the Massachusetts Executive Office of Elder Affairs is currently conducting a demonstration with support from the Robert Wood Johnson Foundation to stimulate use of assistive devices among clients in the Massachusetts state-funded home-care program. The demonstration is providing case managers with training about simple low-cost devices that may help their clients. Case managers are being encouraged to identify clients likely to be receptive to the devices, consult with clients to identify devices potentially helpful to clients, supply the devices, and encourage clients to make use of them. For the Massachusetts program, the use of assistive devices is not new. Case managers have had authorization all along to introduce assistive devices. What is new in the demonstration is the explicit emphasis that is placed on seeking promising applications and encouraging use of the devices.

Expectations for the gains that can be achieved through more extensive use of assistive devices should be realistic. The dramatically lower rates of institutionalization and cost savings reported by Ruchlin and Morris (1981) with the use of personal response systems are very unusual. For the most part, modest contributions are far more likely. More often, assistive devices are likely to permit small reductions in the personal assistance effort that is required. Since most personal assistance is provided by family members, it is they rather than formal services for whom care demands are likely to be diminished. If the gains in reduced personal assistance demands are experienced by family members, the introduction of assistive devices will not lead to a reduction in expenditures for formal services. While assistive devices may permit some reductions in effort required for some forms of personal assistance, it may lead to increases in other areas. Caregivers, for example, may be called upon to set up assistive devices, provide training in their use, and take care of maintenance of the devices. Caregivers may also find themselves shifting the nature of their interaction with care recipients. Caregivers may spend less time performing certain personal assistance tasks but more time providing companionship and supporting expressive activities. For the disabled, assistive devices may lead to quality of life gains more than to reduced reliance on personal assistance. The quality of life gains are likely to be highly specific to the devices and the self-care domains they address. A redesigned and reequipped kitchen, for example, may lead to the preparation of more varied food and result in greater enjoyment of eating. But it may not lead to any change in nutritional intake or to any desired weight change. Further, greater appreciation of food may have no implications for outcomes in any other self-care activity. The use of a variety of assistive devices that effectively address a range of disabilities may lead to an improvement in overall morale. An improvement in morale should not, however, be required to justify the introduction of assistive devices.

This plea for realism in setting expectations for assistive devices in long-term care does not diminish the importance of assistive devices. They represent one of a set of helpful strategies to address the needs of those with disabilities. They are best conceived as complements to other strategies.

CHAPTER 7 　✻　 *Potential Roles for Volunteers*

THE USE OF volunteers for home care has become a minor sub-text in the debate about reducing public spending and controlling agency costs in an era of reduced income and debt reduction. It is also an article of belief for many who are interested in retaining the tradition of family and charitable responsibility. With so many people interested in volunteer activity, why not ask them to take over some of the agency tasks now performed by paid staff, especially for the functionally handicapped. While the evidence is strong that volunteering is still popular, it is not clear that it can take on significant and demanding tasks in home care. In this chapter we will discuss what is known.

Reliance on unpaid volunteers for many community functions has long been an article of faith in America. As early as 1644, Rhode Island recorded a town meeting at which the townspeople promised to come in and help forward the work, which was "to build a small house for old John Mott," who, for thirteen years, "was cared for by 5 different householders with money the town appropriated as necessary for his keeping." Volunteers have been an extension of the family through a larger concept of community help from neighbors and friends. This close connection suggests that the potential for volunteering is influenced by whether the purpose is to save public spending or to help to be of service. Is personal relationship or social responsibility the incentive?

As urbanization and industrialization spread, communities adapted to social change by developing formal and organized health and social agencies which took over much of the mutual helping with philanthropic and tax funds used to employ full-time staff. That staff gradually became professional, developed with financial support from government as well as from community charity campaigns. Volunteering changed as well. In the late nineteenth and early twentieth century many nonprofit associations and corporate entities were staffed by volunteers (usually concerned housewives or unmarried daughters of middle-class families).

Decline and Renewed Interest in Volunteerism

As volunteers were replaced by professional staff, agencies found that limited funding made continued volunteer labor a useful although minor part of the growing service sector. Volunteers became members of governing boards of nonprofit agencies. They ran fundraising campaigns to supplement public funding and performed supplementary staff jobs to release paid staff time for their basic service for clients and the needy. Funding for professional staff continued to grow exponentially between 1945 and 1980, largely as a result of the great increase in public financing for social welfare services. Volunteer efforts became marginal to the basic services. Formal agencies preferred full-time paid staff.

Since 1980, with increased pressure to limit public funding for welfare, organized attention to volunteering has increased as one way to manage the shortfall in financing and to meet the growing interest in home-care services. On the surface this seems especially attractive for the relatively new field of home care and to the emerging assisted living facilities. Its attractiveness is due in part to its close relation to the history of families' caring for their own members. The attitude has survived as family care was supplemented by growing interest in mutual aid through community caring.

Potentials for and Realities of Volunteerism

Numerous national organizations have emerged to promote the value of volunteers—the Association for Volunteer Administration, the National Volunteer Center, the Association for Research in Nonprofit Organizations and Voluntary Action, the Senior Companion Program, Foster Grandparent Program, Retired and Senior Volunteer Program, Points of Light Foundation, the United Way of America, the Salvation Army, and many others. Since 1980 public officials have increasingly urged that churches and other philanthropic organizations, as well as individual citizens contribute more of their time and money to replace a shrinking base of federal tax support for services. Some of this effort is premised on a belief that mutual aid can revitalize a sense of community as responsibilities devolve from Washington to other sectors of society. It may also strengthen the nation's moral stature.

Volunteering in the 1990s

Evidence from several large-scale studies is varied, since definitions of volunteering differ. Most of them find volunteering in general to be widespread. A

Commonwealth Foundation study of a national sample of 2,999 older Americans found that 26 percent of those over 55 did some volunteering. Projected to the entire population, this would represent over 38 million volunteers (Caro and Bass 1995). A 1981 study found 12.6 million people over 55 volunteering. Studies that estimate the value of time spent in volunteering in the economy find that it ranges from $88 billion to $102 billion (Coleman and Kiefer 1986; Morgan 1983).

The Commonwealth Fund Productive Aging Study provides a basis for differentiating among the contributions of those 55 years of age and older as providers of help to their children and grandchildren, as informal caregivers to the sick and disabled, and as volunteers for organizations. When both rates and intensity of involvement with the three types of unpaid assistance are considered, respondents to the nationally representative sample reported the least effort in volunteering for organizations. Including all respondents whether or not they had children, 42 percent reported helping children and grandchildren, typically for six hours per week; 29 percent assisted the sick and disabled, typically for five hours per week; 26 percent volunteered for organizations, typically for 4 hours per week. Particularly striking were the differences in the extent to which the assistance involved substantial time commitments. Of those who helped children and grandchildren, 24 percent did so for 20 or more hours per week; of those who helped the sick and disabled, 19 percent gave assistance for 20 or more hours a week. In the case of volunteering for organizations, only 8 percent contributed 20 or more hours per week (Caro and Bass 1995).

These gross figures may be both exaggerated and underestimated at the same time. Overall, volunteers contribute an average of 4 hours a week but not necessarily every week. Perhaps as many as 900,000 persons over 55 volunteer at least a few hours time in a formal agency; 19 percent average 160 hours annually (Morris and Caro 1996; Herzog and Morgan 1993). The overall figures are impressive but happen to combine help by grandparents and relatives for their own families with help to strangers as a community service. If help to relatives is segregated, by analysis of a different data base, we find that half of those who volunteer help relatives with small children; half do so for an hour a day; those who help disabled relatives do so for an average of 3 hours a week.

From these data it would be concluded that volunteers are looking after a minor segment of need outside the family. Although there is inadequate quantitative evidence, anecdotal evidence is abundant that church groups and neighborhood secular organizations or plain neighborly helping may be more extensive but still limited to members of primary association groups of one kind or another. We do not know how far this extends to "helping the stranger," the touchstone of an ancient religious precept. Nor is the evidence very clear about the content of help given within affinity groups. Is it limited to giving spiritual comfort? Or does it involve maintaining human contact, and performing instrumental tasks like shopping or transporting to a day-care center or a medical clinic? (Morris 1995).

The data to build on is further limited by evidence that the dropout, or "burnout," rate among volunteers is high.

The Needs of a Home-Care Population

When we turn to the real needs of a home-care service, the applicability of known data to expanding services delivered into the home with some combination of volunteer and/or paid staff, the situation is also unclear. For example, client or patient needs at home are becoming increasingly complex as hospitals limit their services to the acute episode and nursing homes are increasingly pressed to serve the more ill who need hospital type professional care. Care at home can demand forms of nursing care, substantial skilled help with personal assistance tasks of movement, dressing, and toilet as well as those instrumental tasks of shopping and cooking or cleaning. Traditionally it has been assumed that nursing or specialist staff can visit a home at intervals to "train someone else at home" to provide the personal assistance required.

The very limited research evidence is that a few relatives will perform such unpleasant tasks at great personal sacrifice; that when demands increase, relatives withdraw (Eggert et al. 1977); and the same happens with neighbors or friends who willingly come in during a crisis but cannot stay for the long term.

As long as the policy trend is to reduce costs, to concentrate more complex cases in medical type institutions, and to try to keep severely disabled persons in their own homes, then the comparative costs of transferring care formerly provided in an institution to the patient's home could end up raising the costs at home closer to those of an institution. Then the policy choice is whether to spend similar per capita sums in an institution or for home care. That becomes a matter of professional and patient preference rather than cost saving, unless the home care costs for sufficient care at home exceed that in an institution.

There are few if any significant studies about how and where the borderline should be drawn. But the experience of Montefiore Hospital in New York City in the 1930s is instructive. That hospital developed a home-care program designed to bring to the home all services (except surgeries, controlled diagnostic studies, etc.) that had been given in the hospital. It established that home delivery was possible, including the medical and personal social supports necessary.

Efforts to expand the idea were, in the long run, frustrated by the fear of public officials that the subsidized costs of a new service would be too great, especially with the risk that family care might be reduced.

In the succeeding years, the complexity of medical care for the severely ill also increased and became more and more costly, keeping alive patients who would once have died but now survived with more complex care needs. What has not been systematically evaluated is whether the greatly escalating hospital and nursing home costs are now such that a comparison of increased cost for care at home would be more favorable for home care. If that were tested anew, we would still face the question whether volunteers, including family members, can take up serious tasks consistently.

If, and it remains a large if, volunteers and family could perform the tasks as part of the redistribution of care responsibilities, would they do so and under what conditions?

In sum, volunteering to do home care needs to be approached with a critical and analytic eye just as much as with a philosophical or ideological commitment to volunteers as one binding force toward community.

The Limitations of Volunteerism—Can They Be Overcome?

It is important to differentiate unpaid help given by a close relative to a family member from that expected to be given by a stranger or friend. Family members perform much of the reported volunteer work. For them, the issue is, How many can do the more demanding tasks on a consistent basis and for how much time daily and weekly?

We use the term *significant volunteering*, or *intensive volunteering*, to differentiate the home-care challenge from the more traditional view of a family with neighborly help doing what families once did in simpler times. For contemporary purposes, we ask whether there are sufficient families whose members can devote nearly full time, say 15–30 hours a week to the personal care of a relative. Or what unrelated individuals would like to volunteer, willing to work that long, consistently, performing difficult personal-care tasks for which they may be trained by a professional. And would their performance be acceptable to the patient, patient's family, and to the training and backup health agency that would have to continue consistent backup services in the home or institution?

The answer is—no one knows, but it is worth testing and may prove feasible. By present evidence, the substitution effect for paid staff will be very limited and may cost more in administration than is saved in payroll.

The Volunteer Pool

The pool of available volunteers is now much reduced from previous years: (1) the one-time charitably minded housewife is more likely to have a full-time job along with spouse, if there is one; (2) families are smaller and adult children all have careers and families of their own; (3) older relatives who retire earlier (often at 55 but surely at 60 or 65) and likely to be in relatively good health for 15–20 years are a major untapped resource, but their willingness is not established; (4) the poor who might have been helpers in the past are now pressed to enter the labor market to work for wages; (5) youth of school age have sometimes been mobilized to help others but their time is limited, and their willingness is usually based on family values of helping others. Anecdotal evidence from colleges report that college youth who had close attachments to their grandparents were most ready to volunteer helping the elderly.

So the pool is greatly reduced, except for the "young old" in group 3 above. The limited evidence from surveys of volunteering thus far indicate that *given the present structure of formal home-care agencies and the rewards* only a few of the retirees are very promising recruits. Most of them want to help but not for heavy duty, meaning most "dirty tasks of personal care," nor for long hours, nor for every week throughout the year. Most want to do something useful mixed with their enjoyment of leisure and search for new experiences. Still a small percentage, 8 percent, already contribute 20 hours or more a week of volunteer time (Caro and Bass 1995). Whether this proportion can be increased awaits restructuring of the service agencies' willingness to experiment with volunteer staff and to turn over significant functions to them. This has usually been considered inefficient use of staff time, risky for clients, and strongly resisted by paid staff and unions in the formal agency system.

Agency and Paid Staff Structural Problems

The expanded use of volunteers requires a major shift in formal agency thinking. Agencies have grown, locally, by relying on paid staff, using volunteers on committees, or performing unchallenging and routine white-collar support functions. Paid staff and unions have a problem with transferring their functions to unpaid staff. Agencies have begun, here and there, to think about how to mix paid and unpaid staff better, especially when the unpaid component is likely to consist of older, though vigorous, persons.

The University of Massachusetts has been experimenting with an elder leadership model that enlists mature adults to make extensive commitments as volunteer coordinators assisting councils on the aging in addressing the needs of the frail elderly. Participants agree to serve 20 hours per week for 45 weeks. They receive training in volunteer coordination and are placed in organizations that need assistance in enlisting and deploying volunteers. The participants develop new volunteering projects. They recruit, train, and support volunteers of all ages who provide various forms of assistance to the frail elderly. The participants receive a modest living allowance. The program was introduced with funding from the Corporation for National Service through the AmeriCorps framework. The project illustrates that it is possible in a carefully organized project to elicit significant volunteer contributions from some older people in a home-care context.

Persisting ethnic differences are also complicating although great progress has been made to overcome some secular and religious barriers. Still there are patient and family discomforts on the side of minorities and of whites when it comes to entrusting one's home to someone from a very different culture. One side may be suspicious about being not respected or being exploited; the other may experience fear and mistrust. Rigorous screening investigations are costly and outside the social welfare agency tradition. While nursing homes have had a great leveling influence, many of them are still effectively segregated by place of residence and are often located in dangerous neighborhoods. Home care, which is often staffed by minorities, bears the weight of a past history of demeaning treatment of minority helpers as ignorant or incompetent maids.

The upward mobility aspirations of minority populations also make personal care of another seem to be a demeaning role without possible career advancement, and this inhibits participation in the volunteer effort by minority youth. Of course, the national drive to move all low-income populations into wage employment is also a major deterrent for younger potential volunteers, especially those offered stipends.

An alternative form of subsidized volunteering is represented by the federally supported Senior Companion Program and Foster Grandparent Program, both of which provide modest stipends ($2.45 per hour) for low-income older persons willing to work 20 hours a week helping homebound elderly persons or at-risk and abandoned children living in hospitals, shelters, and other institutions. Together, these two national senior service programs enable approximately 35,800 older volunteers to help physically and mentally disabled persons in need of assistance. Volunteering with financial incentives clearly works for some. Others interested in volunteering have said they think any work should receive some return. The cost-to-effectiveness ratio has not been measured adequately by outcome standards of self-care, prevention, quality, and cost. The more basic question, in an era of income constraint, is whether other rewards are possible. Aside from public recognition many volunteers report that they would be more enthusiastic if the tasks were clearly important, rather than minor marginal ones.

What Next?

Such analysis leads to the conclusion that volunteering *may* have a significant role in the future. The consumer demand for care at home is likely to increase. At the same time, cost concerns will push against the still uncontrolled rise in spending by hospitals and nursing homes. Furthermore, alternative ways to cope with long-term care needs by more acceptable but cost effective means plus changing consumer expectations are likely to evolve and compete with each other (Morris and Caro 1995).

It will be necessary for home care, as an industry or a field, to attack the manpower questions and the volunteer hopes in some systematic way for the home-care system. We suggest that the most promising path for the future requires the home-care field to examine how best to meet the needs of three different populations. First, one population consists of those with moderate personal-care needs but substantial instrumental needs such as cleaning, transportation, cooking, shopping, and social contact where there are no effective family associations available. Volunteers may find this group most attractive to justify their giving substantial amounts of uncompensated time. Second, another population are those where family members are accessible, or where clients are members (or can become members) of primary affinity groups that offer significant member support. While volunteers may be effective here, some professional concentration will be necessary to tackle the difficult issue of family responsibility for very ill members. It may also involve further work to test whether affinity group members are able to assume what others might view as a family, or a paid staff responsibility—either in an institution or at home. Third, the population of more seriously ill and handicapped who can (as in the Montefiore demonstrations) be sustained in their own homes but with substantial personal care each day plus extensive medical care along with daily living help. This population is the one most easily diverted to an institution, even when the organizational and professional technologies are available to provide effective care at home. For this group the issue is twofold: Can volunteers perform such tasks? And is it cost- and quality-competitive with institutional care at least on a case-by-case basis. It should be kept in mind that much of the policy objection to intensive home care is only sometimes based on total case cost and quality of life comparisons.

More often the public cost concern has been based on fear that families would reduce their helping to take advantage of desirable care that relieves them of both a burden and guilt.

It is possible that one model of a home-care agency can manage all three, or that three types of home care may evolve, much as specialization in nursing home care did. A multilevel and multipurpose home-care agency would be more complex to administer than is usual in most nonprofit social agencies. But some form of specialization is one alternative worth considering.

The second and third models would, we believe, need a core of volunteers to perform what we have called intensive volunteer work, meaning difficulty of the tasks that would be required of volunteers and in the amount of time committed each week, at least 20 or more hours a week for long periods of time. About 8–10 percent of older volunteers already put in that much time, but it is not clear how difficult their duties are. What it comes to is that the combination of paid and volunteer staff, working in close-knit teams would be responsible for caring for much more disabled clients at home than is common today.

Whether by some such modelling, or other means, home care for the future will grow and flourish best if it begins now to attend to such structural, organizational, and practical issues as those described below. We suggest an agenda for better use of volunteers but have serious doubt that it will result in dollar savings through substitution for paid staff, although other benefits such as strong community support for home care could result. The agenda includes:

1. Better analysis of the possible pool of volunteers, with concrete community-wide plans for recruitment

2. Testing incentives to attract the declining pools' members into home care, including rewards other than pay

3. Upgrading the professional skill recognition for caring for the sick as volunteers

4. Designing ways to integrate paid staff, stipendiary, and unpaid volunteers by reassignment of tasks and testing ways to ensure both safety and positive client outcomes

5. Recruiting and recognizing volunteers much as has been recommended for paid staff

6. Moving formal agency efforts toward extensive collaboration with affinity group organizations by sharing territory, tasks, standards, and responsibility

for all, but especially for difficult cases such as the unaffiliated and alone, often elderly women, the mentally ill, and others (Morris and Caro 1995).

Above all, service agencies need to review whether they will be actors within available resources (plus volunteers) to increase the opportunity for seriously disabled populations to be served at home. More intensive and specialized care at home is consistent with the general trend in most health agencies. Volunteers can be a valuable part of service agency adaptation to change, but this option needs a change in thinking plus serious testing. This involves a break from past patterns in which difficult cases were almost automatically passed on by social agencies to some institution. While costs may increase, volunteers may help control the rise so that home care remains competitive for limited public funding. That may mean a transfer of some funds from medical to social organizations, as happened in England's reforms of 1970–90, or an assumption of increasing costs for some parts of home care by the medical system. Any such approach will depend on the home-care agency system's capacity to adapt its structure and thinking.

Finally, it places before the home-care field the task of leading in assessing and reversing the recent trend whereby family members assumed that they need have little responsibility for ill family members. If the current national policy to redistribute public responsibilities in some degree continues, it may offer a major creative opportunity for home care to show how a serious need can be met. The home-care system exists on the border between family and social care and that boundary is where change is likely to take place.

These considerations would also place home care in the 1990s stream of major restructuring of all health and social agencies as different systems of service and care are being pulled apart, reassembled by private organizations and by governmental mandate. Although the argument is set in reduced public spending, there is an undercurrent of demand for better and more effective service systems than those on which home care relied. Demonstration that there are more patterns of family, personal, community (that is volunteers), and paid personnel contributions to long-term illness that can be tried and tested would be evidence of renewed creativity and vigor in the what is nostalgically called "community."

Public funds and national policy will always be a part of the community equation, but they will be strengthened if the community components are willing to justify it by their own actions.

CHAPTER 8 ❉ *The Link between Home Care and Medical Services*

𝓗OME-CARE SERVICES for the ill or disabled and hospital-based or clinical health care services have long been engaged in an uncomfortable embrace in which each needs the other, and yet the two are separated by differences in history, personnel, financing, and public understanding about the populations each serves. The relationship has been further complicated by the changing role of families in providing help for both the short-term convalescent and the long-term chronically ill patient.

If we concentrate on the modern era, from the 1930s to the present, four major forces have been at work affecting the relationship—trends that have been rapidly shifting—and efforts to improve the relationship have changed accordingly. The forces for change have been advances in the technology of medical care and its rising cost; increases in the aged population and extended life in the retirement years; revisions in the structure of the family; and changes in expectations.

The responses can be summarized as extending hospital services to home delivery for short periods of posthospital care; coordinating services, mainly by improved communication technologies; improving coordination of noninstitutional services; and integrating medical and social services including pooled funding for health and social services.

The National Commission on Chronic Illness report in 1956 first defined the relationship as one in which patients with long-term chronic ills and continued disability need not only acute medical attention periodically but also, and equally important, extensive and long continuing social support services. At the time the report was issued, acute medical care was rapidly increasing its need for funds, especially from public sources at a time when funds for welfare were changing from Depression needs to new social problems, usually met by means-tested income services for basic maintenance. Health care was accepted as benefiting all citizens; the latter mainly the minority poor needing "charitable" help.

This chapter is a brief review of the various approaches to integrating health (or medical) and social support services, without discussing the results in detail. The purpose is to outline some approaches and then discuss what each of them can mean for the future of home care.

Factors Reshaping Linkage

SCIENCE AND MEDICAL TECHNOLOGY

Until the 1930s, medicine, despite its achievements and long history, had limited technical capacity to prevent or cure disease or to achieve secondary or tertiary prevention. A major boost in capacity to treat and cure occurred with the discovery of antibiotics, which made possible the near-conquest of the pulmonary infections that had previously led to early death for many people in their mature years. This led in part to the increase in numbers of adults surviving into later years. This was called "a failure of success" (Gruenberg 1994) because it led to increased numbers of older citizens succumbing to late life enfeeblement or to incurable chronic ills leading to physical dependence on others.

A dramatic example evolved out of World War II—the technical capacity to help young veterans with spinal cord injury live almost normal lives with the most severe handicaps. Similar achievements followed in saving newborn infants with very low birth weights but high risk of survival with lifelong handicaps. Varied therapies helped those with long-term and handicapping neurological diseases as well as those suffering from severe traumas of industrial, sports, and automobile accidents to function with their disabilities. Technology to intervene in cases of cardiac disease and renal failure, to name only two, also added to the growing list of human ills for which new hope could be promised.

These successes also encouraged increased medical attention to advanced research to find the causes and then the treatments that could prevent many of the remaining chronic and disabling ills. Altogether these developments led the medical system to concentrate on improving what it could not cure and to continue the search for cures and prevention. When complete restoration of function was not possible, long life with disability was still possible, but that challenge involved a variety of social supports and only intermittent access to the medical institution.

The cost of the new technologies, plus the challenge of rapid changes in science, led major medical facilities, under pressure from financing agencies, to contain their costs, leading in turn to the transfer of most long-term care deliverable out of the hospital to the other institutions or to families.

INCREASE IN THE AGED POPULATION
AND LONGER LIFE IN RETIREMENT

The increase in the numbers of feeble elderly and disabled of all ages who needed some support other than active medical treatment increased the demand for alternative and less familiar services. The need was captured by the headline "What to Do When the Doctor Leaves" (Morris 1973). The major resource continued to be the family, which in turn was changing. Mothers and wives stayed in the workforce after World War II or entered it when they could. Nursing homes and homes for the aged were traditional solutions that encountered changes in public expectations and were increasingly costly as their applicants began to need more physical and social care and as their life expectancy lengthened.

Care delivered to the home became an alternative resource. It was rooted in a welfare system for the poor, subsidized by public funds—homemakers for the aged and public health nurses or visiting nurses for the sick and for poor mothers with newborn infants. With enactment of Medicare and Medicaid in 1965 visiting nurse services and public welfare were pushed to extend their prior short-term welfare homemaker and educational services to long-term care (Phillips 1971). Between 1961 and 1971 the number of homemaker agencies of all kinds grew from 208 to 1800, employing 20,000 homemakers.

CHANGES IN THE STRUCTURE OF THE FAMILY

The family continued to be a major resource, but it too was changing. Women entered the workforce and family size decreased. There were fewer family members at home, out of the labor force, to look after a handicapped relative. Further, rising expectations about a better life for all put three-generation families in a squeeze between doing more for their children and more for aged relatives. Where incomes were large, services could be purchased privately. But with median incomes at between $25,000, then rising to $35,000 (often with two adults working) this solution was beyond the reach of more than half the population.

CHANGING EXPECTATIONS

More than family expectations about what modern society could assure them has been the change in public perception about institutional care. Mental hospitals, chronic disease hospitals, and, more recently, nursing homes came to be viewed as unmanageably costly in human as well as dollar terms. Scientific progress pulled in its wake a belief that social technology could do as well—that institutions should be reserved for a relatively few conditions requiring full-time skilled nursing and medical attention. Most handicapped, whether for psychological or physiological reasons, could live in homes of their own (or of their families) with medication and social supports. This peaked in the deinstitutionalization of the mentally ill with public support in the 1963 Community Health Centers on the assumption that mental health centers could manage the treatment of most mentally ill and mentally retarded while they lived at home. Failure was due to a combination of erratic funding and professionally misplaced priorities. Social support services suited to the new care at home were not funded (Knee and Lamson 1971).

Slowly, a growing number of agencies tried to meet these challenges, caring for people with chronic and often terminal conditions—cancer, the progressive neurological diseases—whose needs extended to months and years, in slow progression. But the boundaries began to blur about which agencies would finance services during these long-term disabilities or illnesses.

Responses to the Need for Linkage

THE HOSPITAL-BASED HOME-CARE APPROACH

As early as the 1930s, Montefiore Hospital experimented with a home-care service to deliver anything the hospital staff could perform (except surgery) to a patient discharged to his or her own home. It soon included social supports if those were found to be necessary. It was intended at first to take care of post-hospital short-term needs, much like accelerated convalescent care, as good for the patient and for the hospital's budget. But as the demands extended into long-term care, the program had to be drastically modified.

A medical home care service had been started by the Boston University Medical Center in the nineteenth century, but it was limited to sending student interns and nurses into the home as part of their medical education.

In the 1960s hospital-based home care was tried by many hospitals, but it usually resulted in small-scale demonstrations for short periods of posthospital care at home built around physicians and nurses as well as social workers and aides. The Veterans Administration (see chap. 5) introduced its aid and attendance program for chronic care and a long-term community foster home program for recovered alcoholics. The aid and attendance program used both family and foster residences while the successful home-care program for addictions used group homes in a hospital's region. In both cases, hospital social work and nursing staff were used to check the home and inform family or foster family members about care needed. The hospital guaranteed quick response in case of any medical or behavioral emergency, including immediate hospital preadmission when needed.

The extensive New York City public hospital program also adopted home-care programs and was the only hospital-based system that served several thousand discharged patients in their own homes and continued to do so for years. Unique conditions in New York may have made this expansion possible; its large numbers of minority families, where care within the family continued as a tradition, helped, but they could do so only with supportive social services given their desire for work opportunities out of the home and rising expectations about quality of life: New York developed the most extensive home-care program in the nation for Medicaid eligible patients, which accounted for over 50 percent of all care at home for 35,000 patients a year, for an average of 50 hours of service a week. This was backed by a unique state constitution that mandated that "care be provided for the needy."

After the initial interest, pressure to contain medical costs became dominant. Hospital-based home care became at best an extension of medical services, and financing was limited to short-term posthospital care while active treatment was completed. It has seldom been possible to draw on medical funds for expanded social services for personal assistance to support long-term medical care outside the hospital.

Instead of managing home care, most hospitals developed discharge programs staffed by nurses or social workers to help family members plan the care of a patient about to be discharged. This included counseling and helping the family anticipate what it needed to do. If the postmedical care needs were likely to be long term or complex, the discharge staff could only rely on other agencies, often with limited resources. The discharge function was mainly to have patients out of the hospital quickly. In most cases the family received information and was left to arrange what it could. Home visits by nurses or therapists were provided only as long as hospitals and doctors were actively treating the patients.

This very limited attempt to link the hospital to social services grew in response to pressures on hospitals to reduce length of patient stay to move chronic cases out quickly, as a way to limit hospital costs. But small discharge staffs could reach only a fraction of handicapped patients before they were discharged and staff authority was very limited.

The introduction of prospective payment, by which hospitals were reimbursed by insurers only for services and care identified as the average for an area, may have accelerated the transfer to out-of-hospital providers of care. As a budget control it did not address the fact that the early days of hospitalization are the most costly. Patients who were discharged earlier often needed both medical care to complete a course of treatment plus functional supports at home. These had been absorbed during the in-hospital stay. It did have the effect of transferring patients who were likely to be more ill in the early days of their return home as well as those who, historically, had been kept in hospitals for long periods of time because of hard-to-manage chronic illness. (It is difficult to recall the time when, prior to 1940, it was not uncommon for some hospitals to serve both the acute and the chronic patient under one administration, although with different degrees of staff and facility investment. Affluent or influential patients could then be kept in hospital for weeks and months.)

The hospital discharge system had one further limitation. Its social service department usually heard about and served patients with limited incomes, those likely to be uninsured or in receipt of some welfare. The great proportion of hospital patients were not indigent. They came in and left through their family doctor, who rarely had a complete understanding about or responsibility for the care of patients after hospitalization. A few teaching hospitals such as Beth Israel in Boston made serious efforts to inform medical students and residents. Slowly physicians acquired some understanding about the social needs of long-term patients, but the pace of hospital discharges made it difficult for understaffed discharge departments to keep up with most discharged patients.

In a few teaching hospitals there was a short-lived movement to instruct physicians to perform the follow-up planning of their patients. In effect this would have replaced some of the need for social work counseling of families in a medical system if, and only if, physicians could perform both medical and social counseling. This concept surfaced, in limited form, in the social and health maintenance organization and PACE (On Lok) experiments discussed below (Cohen, Kumar, and McGuire 1991).

An experiment in England in the early 1970s encouraged small groups of physicians to share an office and to employ, with subsidy, a social worker to perform the linking task for the group practice. Something like this later emerged as some health maintenance organizations, under the pressure for managed care, began to employ a social worker or nurse consultant.

Home-care agencies now depend on a variety of sources for their clientele, and among them hospitals are important. But this has not led to any significant enrichment of the seamless web theory for long-term care. Agencies are a safety valve for hospitals that need or want to reduce length of stay. The service agency receives limited information. There was some opportunity to integrate both medical and social services through referrals back and forth, but there is little continuity of staff or data experience and little functional information exchanged about most disabled patients. Clients are not often directly involved when social service staff in each agency exchange views by telephone, mail, or case conferences. Hospital practices are little altered in managing chronic disability except as physicians become familiar with the discrete social services available. Social agencies slowly adapt their services, and their staffs learn about some medical conditions. Since the direction is governed by each referring hospital's needs and understanding, the agency usually continues in its usual pattern of delivering a specific social service without entering far into the hospital culture or bringing the medical culture into its work.

Coordinating the Medical and Community Social (Home-Care) Services

More extensive coordinating efforts were expanded after the 1960s and especially in the 1970s to improve the linkage between medical and community services. These were less system building and more based on new communications technology. In several sites major public funds were invested in setting up electronic systems. Some maintained databases about the wide range of services in the community, eligibility, extremely varied costs, and applications procedures. These were intended to give workers in any agency, including medical ones, as well as patients and their families or friends, easy access to the sources of help to which they could turn.

These data sources served many purposes but did not solve the linkage problem for many reasons. Social service systems need information about a patient, but hospitals seldom commit to public access useful data about a patient other than a diagnosis and date of service. Furthermore, the readmissions to hospitals reported by home-care social or nursing services in case of emergency are not easy to access fast enough to fit a new medical model of community-based care. The shortage of home-care services leads to waiting lists, especially for personal assistance. A service listing does not mean availability. And varying eligibility rules change frequently. In the end the databases give a map of a maze, but anyone seeking to link the pieces must go through an arduous search and negotiation task to fit pieces together. The medical system lacks the patience or resources, and quick response is needed. The valid concern over privacy of patient information means that necessary information is often missing. Physicians are seldom specific about the kind of *functional* service their patients need and often lack clear understanding about functional limitations. And social agencies, being rooted in a welfare and means-tested tradition, seldom commit to accepting a case without their own investigation of ability to pay. The exceptions to these problems are that minority of patients with ample means to pay full fees without question.

The result is that the two different systems still rely upon staff-to-staff negotiations over each complicated case or on organizational negotiation to develop community plans and responsibilities that take time to settle the arrangement of financing. This approach has the advantage of bringing different providers together on behalf of complex cases. It also brings to the surface gross service deficiencies but the providers have no authority to act on remedying them. Over time, the testimony about need has some effect on planning but not in time for the needs of patients caught between two separate systems.

For a time a movement to bring most service agencies or their branches together under one roof called colocation was popular. It did make life easier for staff and for quick personal negotiation. It had the disadvantage of centralization, which meant that the access point was less accessible for the patient.

Coordination has little direct influence on changing the functioning of a social agency. It is a means for making each service more efficient by reducing unnecessary duplication of effort, by improving access to existing services, by sharing and exchanging referrals, and by identifying communitywide needs for social services or for changes in medical care. This can result as staffs add up their individual experiences to strengthen community support to fill unmet needs in the social welfare and in medical provision. But the process is not quick and results often haphazard. The needs of the medical and welfare systems are not easily modified in the direction of medical and social integration. Not many medical centers have created geriatric or disability specialty centers that combine clinical care and attention to at-home care.

An Integrated System?

For many years advocates of home care, especially long-term home care, have urged an integrated system that could provide "a seamless, comprehensive, web of services for all ages." This idea has been generally accepted, but there have seldom been efforts to translate the concept into practice. Since the 1970s there have been at least two approaches: expanding the reach of medical concepts to a vertical and horizontal integration of services and small but significant research and development projects supported by the Health Care Finance Administration.

In the 1980s, experiments in social and health maintenance organizations

(SHMOs), and in PACE (On Lok) among others, have tried to fuse physician, nursing, and social services into one administrative and capitated system. In each case, a variety of community services are necessary, but the core of the system begins with a unified structure in which the therapeutic and social support services are at least planned for and financed.

The SHMO was authorized by Congress to test capitation payment for an insured population for medical, hospital, nursing home, *and* social support services, including physical or occupational therapy, to show that it can work (Leutz, Greenlick, and Capitman 1994). The rate is set at 100 percent, rather than 95 percent of the average adjusted per capita costs for other HMOs. The provider is at full or limited risk to provide all that is promised within the capitation. The intent is for physicians treating a patient to have an incentive to use community services in place of much more costly medical or hospital or nursing home care whenever it is deemed appropriate. An estimated 22,000 patients were enrolled initially.

PACE (On Lok), also with congressional authority, has extended to several sites. It is based on Medicaid reimbursement primarily and is limited to severely handicapped patients living at home who are nursing home eligible but want to stay at home. They also agree to abide by the plan rules. These include use of a specified hospital and primary care medical team; agreement to come several times a week to a day care center. Hospitalization, some drugs, and all other costs are covered. The reimbursement rate is generous. There is no clear conclusion about how broadly the plan could be extended to a less selective population or whether its costs will remain competitive as new programs evolve. An estimated 2700 patients were enrolled in experimental sites in 1996 (U.S. Senate 1996).

There were other experiments but these are the clearest examples of an attempt to integrate medical and social, acute and long-term services in a medical model. The SHMO results are especially useful because they serve a population at many income levels and all ages. The PACE results are equally useful for a narrower population.

The SHMO experiment worked through an HMO funded by private insurance, private fees, or Medicare reimbursement for a population over 65. Beginning with 4 sites, then growing to 8, with one dropping out, its integration took place in Medicare-approved contracts to medical HMOs authorized to enroll members under insurance contract guaranteeing the delivery of Medicare benefits, drugs, ancillary services plus up to $1000 a month for community long-term care and for short-term nursing home care. The enrolled population is carefully managed to limit the proportion of enrollees with severe health problems in order to avoid adverse selection. An average sum per enrollee is guaranteed the HMO for all services delivered. The HMO is at risk to live within the reimbursed amount for the experimental population.

The HMO physician and staff make decisions with their patients. Every effort is made to encourage staff to use alternative social services at home and to reduce hospital or nursing home use. At the same time care has been evaluated to see whether the covered population benefited in health outcomes and whether the overall costs compared favorably with conventional fee-for-service financing (Leutz and Greenlick 1994; Leutz 1995).

The evaluation of results has been difficult, and there are differing interpretations about outcomes. There seems to have been an increase in the use of community services compared with other medical practices. The evaluation took place after only three years of experience, a short time for testing so complex a system. The critics and the proponents differ in both evaluative methodologies used and in conclusions (Leutz 1995).

On balance it is clear that the SHMOs that have persisted and increased their experimental sites from 4 to 8 are convinced that a basic redesign in health care delivery is in the making. The PACE (On Lok) sites have also been increased and depend on public financing to a large extent. The critics have argued that healthier patients in SHMO do very well but that the very frail do not. The differences, however, may be a matter of methodologic semantics. For example, the proponents argue that a system that frequently evaluates enrollee health status catches changes in the functional status of individuals early and moves them into a higher risk population more quickly. This encourages early treatment, even though the result, statistically, appears to suggest that the healthy are better off because the more sick are removed from the group for reporting purpose, to a group more risky and handicapped.

The arguments over technical measurements do not undermine the claims made but do reveal a serious and long-standing problem in health care—the separation of scientific interest for the more healthy from the already chronically sick or handicapped. The SHMOs argue that under any system of health care, older handicapped patients of any age require more time from providers; it is unrealistic to expect that a combined medical and social system will alter the physiological realities of deteriorating health conditions not due to neglect or delay in treatment. Unfortunately, the emphasis on cost savings has made it difficult to establish just when and how spending more, or less, clearly produces longer life or earlier death or less handicap rather than more. The evaluations of this model have not settled the matter.

For our purposes the experience makes clear that closely linking prescription and financing for an integrated medical and social service system is easier to argue for conceptually than it is to carry out in a world where cost is an overpowering consideration.

The experiments do, however, suggest the value of a few lessons.

1. Long-term care does require its own standards, which differ from those for the healthier or more able patient.

2. An insurance approach designed for an aged population (Medicare eligible) needs to refresh its membership constantly with younger enrollees so that the most at-risk patients do not remain as the population ages, something not easy to do without universal health insurance to spread risks over a broader population base to start with.

3. It is not clear yet how well these experiments incorporate personal assistance at home.

While there are benefits from this experimental fusion, it raises some doubt whether managed care for the long-term patient is best developed from a geriatric base as is argued by those who propose to expand Medicare entitlement. A separate geriatric design may be necessary if funding is from sources committed only to the population over 65, in order to account for the differences in time necessary per patient and the greater prevalence of disability and chronic illness, despite the concomitant improvement in the health of the younger retired. But such solutions do not yet answer the question: How well can a medicine-based system agree to meet long-term personal assistance needs?

This would seem to leave unsettled the arguments in favor of a separate long-term care option or benefit, and even begs the question: where does personal assistance fit on the priority totem pole? Should it be part of Medicare or part of a universal health insurance for all ages and all conditions, including the long term. On such issues, home care is either divided, or still on the periphery of that debate.

Like SHMOs, PACE (On Lok) has concentrated on the nursing home eligible population which could be cared for at home. As a model for home care, it concentrates on the poor of any age, dependent on some public assistance since it is financed by Medicaid. It does offer to combine medical treatment with a required regular use of at least one type of social service, adult day care. Its results are no less unsettled. It has helped individuals, but these gains have not been evaluated as strictly against a control population. It has been successful in securing congressional support for more demonstration sites, perhaps because of its concentration on a low-income population.

This model offers evidence for some home-care growth but not necessarily for personal assistance that will require more extensive commitment by all agencies to join in such demonstrations than has yet appeared. Lacking that, home care with personal assistance would retain its separate character, being a referral source but subject to changes made by others in the provider marketplace.

Vertically and Horizontally Integrated Systems

Since the 1980s, there has been pressure to move most health care to some form of managed care under competitive conditions, where private (or public) insurers place their contracts with providers offering the lowest cost package of services or offering the most qualitatively attractive package.

Many hospitals have moved quickly to consolidate their competitive positions to assure maximum flow of patients and thus income. There is no standard formula, but in general a major hospital or coalition of hospitals will join forces in one administration and then add to its service panoply, groups of primary care physicians, specialists, rehabilitation agencies, home-care services, day-care centers, transportation services, and ambulatory care centers for surgery and for medicine. The aim is to assure that one administration can, ultimately, control and deliver a wide range of services radiating into and out of the hospital center, which remains the center of most advanced technologies, for training, research, and the like.

These horizontal and local considerations have been accompanied by extensive vertical consolidation with absentee centralized ownership of chains of hospitals. These are mainly for-profit corporations using the strength of large capital resources and aggregated purchasing power to reduce their costs, to force providers to reduce charges, and to negotiate low reimbursement rates. The consequences are not yet clear, but charges of fraudulent billing and exercise of undue economic pressure to force local providers into an absentee corporate controlled system have been levied. Without conclusive experience, the trend has brought health care (with professional and local tradition) into potential conflict with a commercial tradition. McArthur and Moore have discussed the murky territory when two cultures (commerce and professionalism) confront each other in what may become a revolution in health care (McArthur and Moore 1997).

These trends are too new to provide a clear picture of results. It remains to be seen whether such a system can do better in smoothing out the relationships and the patient and staff uses of the various services better than that achieved by independent services with some coordination of their efforts.

There also remains the question of whether the attention of such a system will be focused mainly on the relatively short term after hospitalization or on the preventive aspects of medical plus social services to prevent chronicity and disability at secondary and tertiary levels, as well as at the primary prevention level; whether it will follow patients with long-term needs, mainly social in nature; whether medical dollars, flowing in comparative profusion compared to funding for social services, will be pooled and allocated any differently; whether the system will benefit the more healthy younger population but do less well for the very poor, the uninsured, and populations with genetic and other risks of high-cost medical and support care.

In 1998 it is most likely that these coalitions will produce a new subacute medical system for short periods of postacute, posthospital services—a medical service focused on cure. But it is not clear that the postacute period will give more attention to social support needs than it has in the past. The role of these coalitions can be attractive for short-term home care, but to build its place home care would need to modify its structure to respond to the requirements of such a medical construct. Over time a comprehensive system might evolve, one that might exist under a dominantly private insurance system as well under a public insurance, as is the case today. But will costs to include personal assistance be more acceptable in any of them if they use a medical criterion to allocate resources? With its size, can such an integrated system be flexible and adapt swiftly to new technologies and to fiscal limitations imposed by family choices or by public financial limits?

For the 1990s, the driving force is that of privately insured competitive managed care, which will seek to assimilate the competition pressure through a market to save money while the public demands high-quality care for all conditions and populations. The sheer variety of human health needs of different populations may be well served by such integration or alternatively may need a reexamination of the potentials of specialization that have evolved in the past sixty years.

It is too early to know just how the hospital-centered vertical and horizontal integrations now being formed will play out. On past record, their course will be dominated by the needs of hospitals and of acute care medicine, though now expanded to include "subacute" services for relatively short periods of time, comparable to the one-time convalescent home. If personal assistance home-care agencies could strengthen their role sufficiently to become important to the needs of medical care, they could become influential parts of a new integration, but remain as independent corporations, much as many small producers function as satellite essentials for larger industrial and commercial corporations.

Building a Separate Home- and Community-Based System

While the concept of an integrated health and welfare system for long-term care has long been an objective, the events outlined above have preempted most advocate energies. In the meantime, the social support services for home delivery, rooted mainly in public welfare, continued to develop on their own with substantial means-testing for the poor—for nursing home care and for home-care alternatives.

State departments of human services and other agencies supported in part by funds from the Older Americans Act (OAA), Medicaid, and general revenue encouraged expansion of services for the elderly poor sometimes through publicly administered agencies such as the Home Care Corporations of Massachusetts. These agencies coordinated public funds, and sometimes private funds, to service agencies, for meals on wheels, transportation, visiting nurse and homemaker services, day care, and social programs. Since funds were limited, compared with those for medical care, such agencies for a long time tended to serve the moderately handicapped and ill. With least evidence of improvement, the most handicapped were often considered too costly to justify major home-care investment from limited public funds. This left the seriously handicapped dependent on nursing home care or family help. By the 1980s, most states began to press these agencies to concentrate on the more critically ill populations.

A variety of nonprofit agencies for specific diseases also grew in numbers and influence. Some, such as the Easter Seal Society, offered varied rehabilitation and care service for children, in association with medical facilities. Others raised funds for research and public information about conditions as varied as cancer, Alzheimer's disease, multiple sclerosis, and many more. Their contribution has been to raise political understanding of the need for financial support for people suffering from these diverse conditions. The funds usually were channeled into the existing service agencies noted above. Although these advocates gave eloquent testimony about need, they were unable to agree about changes in the delivery system that could address the deficiencies outlined in other chapters.

Demonstrations and experiment were launched by the Levinson Policy Institute of Brandeis University between 1970 and 1980 to promote the growth in home-delivered services emphasizing social supports and personal attendants. Its early argument was based on the assumed economies if home care was made available as a cost-effective as well as humane alternative to a nursing home. Its demonstrations led in Massachusetts to the home-care corporation, in Wisconsin to the Community Option Program, and to numerous variations such as the Connecticut Triage and the Monroe County, New York programs (see Chapter 1).

These early initiatives were based on welfare payments plus family and community nonprofit cooperation. By 1980 more general funding via Medicare and the Health Care Finance Administration led to other versions. The public concern over rising heath expenditures also led to the introduction of an extensive federal program of waivers issued to states that could produce an acceptable plan to use available public funds (federal and state) administered by the state in flexible ways to divert patients from costly nursing home and unnecessary hospital care to less costly home care. The varieties of state initiatives have been extensive and have not yet been comprehensively catalogued or evaluated. A majority of states have received waiver authority for stimulating new approaches without going through traditional channels of service. Whether justified or not, the formula has been "do more with less." One incentive has been that, with waivers to experiment, states could save some money, which they could then use to expand to hitherto excluded populations. Critics have generally praised the intentions but have produced conflicting evidence about the cost saving promised (Weissert, Cready, and Pawelak 1988).

In the years 1980–96 the various advocacy and service agencies have generally continued to present testimony about unmet needs, each specialty stressing its select population. They have not yet effectively joined forces to develop a different system for long-term care, lobbying mainly for increased funds to be allocated to existing agencies with existing structures.

At this time the options seem to be these: (1) a two-tier system for short periods of acute and postacute care managed by institutions with most advanced technologies and most professional personnel beside long-term personal assistance and social supports managed by the family and means-tested agencies for the poor, which become available to the middle class after they dispose of their assets to become welfare eligible; (2) a consolidated social support system pooling medical and welfare funds and redivision of all funds to embrace both long-term and short-term social help for patients regardless of age.

To develop a freestanding social support home-care system would require extensive rethinking and restructuring as outlined in chapter 12. This has not had much support from home-care advocates, most of whom prefer the seamless web attached to health care, perhaps because it is familiar and associated with the most appealing source of funds in the public eye.

The Managed Approaches: Contracting Out

Since the emergence of privately insured managed care an interesting alternative has emerged, based on the principles of competitive managed care to control costs but offering a new way to meet long-term care needs within that policy. A good example is that of Community Health Associates of Massachusetts, which is also being tested in four states. In this approach a group of physicians and nurse practitioners offer to relieve insurers (and others) of the responsibility of caring for identified seriously handicapped and costly cases such as trauma patients, spinal cord injuries, progressive neurological diseases, AIDS patients, and the like. These are difficult to manage and costly, and insurers seek to avoid such patients if at all possible, as do many providers. The associates offer to negotiate the costs of these patients to insurers and then for a subcontract to assume full responsibility for all services, medical, nursing, social, and so on. They have succeeded in providing more acceptable care to such populations at the negotiated price. The cost to insurers is acceptable since they have to pay for care anyway. The associates staff is adequately compensated and can pay for whatever is needed. Patients seem to be more satisfied with the specialized care they receive and disenrollment is minimal (Master et al. 1996).

The results are possible because of specialized skill in handling all needs by expanded use of nurse practitioners versed in comprehensive long-term care and by maximizing patient and family self-care potentials and careful use of all alternatives. In a health system now based on price and quality competition for patients, the associates offer both price and quality competitively. But whether it argues for more use of speciality nursing or also incorporates social supports in its capitation is not known. Whether the approach can be widely applied will depend on the ability to train physician and nursing staff in the specialized approaches that the group has evolved and whether they can maintain the competitive edge for special cases over the standard service approach.

Such an approach has also been tried in a limited way by some visiting nurse associations (Boston). Nurse practitioners have been admitted to some hospitals to locate patients whom the acute hospital staff has difficulty discharging. The association then proposes to take over the discharge and care of patients it believes it can handle in the community and agrees on the price to transfer care to the association. It can employ its own personal care aides or contract for them. The nursing service assumes some risk, but if its judgment is sound, it has succeeded in securing early discharge of complex cases to community care and succeeded in maintaining them in the community. The numbers have been small and how this could grow is uncertain. But the basic concept is compatible with the managed-care trend. It offers a new way to deal with patient, family, and professional needs and preferences with a capitated payment system.

This approach has been tried in nursing-oriented home health agencies in a small way. For personal assistance home care, it would involve major restructuring in order to develop the ability to manage a category of complex of needs, much as has been the case in the Community Health Associates and SHMO and PACE (On Lok) models. We doubt if this approach is attractive to most agencies rooted in social service. If tried, it could become a major part of a substantial freestanding home-care system as outlined in the concluding chapter.

Conclusion

The relationship between a home service plan requiring substantial active medical care plus major personal assistance and a plan that relies mainly on personal assistance and intermittent services provided by a family physician or registered nurse is ambiguous. The interplay between medical and personal care shifts over the life course of any patient. This schema may help clarify why the shifting responsibilities also confound efforts to simplify financing that treats all components of a care plan equitably. (See fig. 1 in chap. 2.)

Phase 1: Medical services are dominant—managed in a hospital or related health care facility with intensive medical and paramedical care for a condition that is expected to improve or be corrected in a short time. Major financing: public and private health insurance plus some nonprofit and family sharing. Personal assistance is a minor consideration.

Phase 2: Medical and personal care services deliverable at home are therapeutically interdependent and equally necessary but organizationally split for the period in transition to physical restoration. The medical care is covered by an accredited health care agency but is also dependent on provision of personal care at home. Basic financing for the health care component comes from public or private insurance. Coverage of personal care services may be covered but it is dependent on limitations in health insurance policies and medical opinion, which vary considerably. Instead, continued life at home is heavily dependent on (a) close and willing family; (b) a home-care service financed mainly by public or private welfare funds, which are modest; (c) erratic and ambiguous insurance coverage.

Phase 3: Personal assistance at home is dominant. Medical interventions are limited to maintenance and prevention and mainly support the personal care plan at home. The minor medical component is essential, but financing is limited. Organized personal care services are scantily financed by (a) medical insurance, which concentrates on diverting patients from nursing homes or on restrictive definitions attached to the delivery of medical service; (b) various welfare programs for helping the disabled and feeble elderly and some for the younger disabled. The bulk of financing is dependent on family or close neighbor networks and a miscellany of specialized home-care social services.

The link between medical and social services remains important for both systems, but no consensus can be seen about how to optimize it. Many medical and health agencies have added a limited but significant home health care component to their thinking. Most of the shift is governed, properly, by their primary responsibility for the sick. This responsibility has now moved outside the hospital and the doctor's office.

What remains unresolved is Who is *primarily accountable* for the nonclinical services that which are necessary in long-term chronic illness? Medicine is central to health. Isn't personal and social help central to long-term life at home with disability? If the latter is accepted as central too, will it evolve as a support *within* a medical system even when medicine is only intermittently involved? Thus far this seems unlikely. The alternative remains a dilemma. Can a stable social support structure be an independent resource, or must it remain appended to a dominant health system? (See emerging insurance proposals in Chapter 10.)

CHAPTER 9 ❋ *Assisted Living as a Surrogate for the Changing Idea of "Home"*

THE CONCEPT OF assisted living is difficult to translate into a neat typology. Nevertheless, it is increasingly the choice of functionally disabled consumers and their families who are looking at the options available between remaining at home and moving into a nursing home. The circumstances that ordinarily precipitate an investigation of assisted living opportunities arise when individuals develop physical or psychological handicaps that limit their capacity to perform all the functions of daily life; or when they begin to fear that they may become handicapped and want to prepare against that eventuality.

Assisted living can be viewed as a continuously refined series of homelike arrangements augmented by an array of security and personal care services. The emergence of assisted living is thus best viewed as an ongoing effort to increase individual choices and to fit varied service wants and desired life styles together. The attraction of assisted living is that it offers the resident privacy, security, and maximum control over his or her arrangements for obtaining assistance with one or more activities of daily living, for example, eating, dressing, bathing, transferring, toilet, laundry, housekeeping, transportation, and recreation. Light nursing and medical care are specially procured as they are by any person no matter where they live or are provided by contract by the assisted living facility. There is no precise information on the number of assisted living residences in the United States; however, the American Association of Homes and Services for the Aging (AAHSA) reports that estimates taken in 1993 indicate assisted living facilities ranged in number from 30,000 to 40,000 and served an estimated one million older persons (AAHSA 1997; Assisted Living Facilities Association of America 1993).

Defining the Field of Supply

Various attempts have been made to establish a typology of this variety of housing. The Assisted Living Facilities Association of America defines assisted living as "a special combination of housing and personalized health care designed to respond to individual needs of those who need help with activities of daily living" (Kane and Wilson 1993). (Note the ambiguous word "special."). The American Health Care Association defines assisted living as "a residential setting that provides or coordinates personal care services, 24-hour supervision and assistance, activities, and health-related services, and is designed to minimize the need to move and maximize privacy and independence." Kane, in a report to the American Association of Retired Persons (AARP), proposed "any *group* residential program that is not licensed as a nursing home, that (usually) provides (individualized) personal care to persons with need for assistance in the activities of daily living and that can respond to unscheduled needs for assistance that might arise" (Kane and Wilson 1993). The AARP proposed a new supra category, "supportive housing," which includes several subtypes.

1. Board and care homes: group residences that provide room and board, 24-hour protective supervision and assistance with some daily living requirements. The term includes homes for the aged and residential health care facilities.

2. Assisted living: group residences that add to the provisions in board and care homes; they "tend to be more upscale, usually providing private rooms with baths or small apartments, social and recreational opportunities."

3. Adult foster care: room and board, with varying levels of supervision and assistance with daily living requirements; they are generally small and family-run with an emphasis on maintaining a family atmosphere.

4. Continuing care retirement communities (CCRCs): hotel-style services to all residents with a guarantee of some level of personal and health care (Sherwood et al. 1997).

5. Congregate housing: private living quarters with meals in a central facility and shared common spaces.

6. Centers for independent living: programs that combine medical assistance, personal assistance, and other social supports, mainly for severely handicapped younger adults and veterans (White et al. 1996).

There can be quibbling about such attempts to introduce some order into the subject. For example, homes for the aged may object to being included with board and care homes since many offer a wide range of services. And "residential health care facilities" could include nursing homes, which may consider themselves much closer to a medical facility.

More important is the exclusion of the usual family home of most potential consumers. If the space to be filled includes the above types of housing as "supportive," the exclusion of public housing, of condominia, as well as the conventional freestanding home is worth keeping mind. This much larger housing market is also changing and home-care services delivered to this market do not differ much from home care delivered under contract to an assisted-living complex. The key difference is in the extent of control transferred by the consumer to a management entity of some kind. In the end it is possible that consumer choices will decide supply. Demand may be determined not only by refinements in services offered but also by the extent to which consumers may or may not wish to transfer control when they face some limited physical or emotional handicap.

Another defining factor in consumer choice as the options are expanded is the divide between single adults and couples. Much of the search for alternative living arrangements comes from individuals living alone with a scanty support circle of friends or family. Married couples have the choice of support if one spouse is handicapped and the other able to help. While these choices are not at all clear cut, they are part of the problem in defining whence comes the demand. All of these service variations have constantly tried to improve both the scope and complexity of their offerings and also to make facilities more like a home than an institution. These facilities constantly try to improve privacy arrangements and more complex services dependent on more professional staff and technology to help the disabled to live relatively independent lives. At the same time consumer expectations about quality of life and freer access to new services have improved, while concern about rising costs persist.

A Financing Classification

Callahan (1996) has proposed a model derived mainly from financing alternatives: (1) private insurance; (2) Medicare; (3) Medicaid; (4) naturally organized retirement communities; (5) social health maintenance organizations (SHMOs); (6) state-run case management programs, usually for Medicaid eligible or low-income groups; (7) private and often proprietary assisted living with management company and resident negotiated benefits; (8) Pace/On Lok for nursing home eligible.

Source of financing is an important consideration for most programs. Will they survive only with private pay residents and how long can residents afford to pay? What are the rules governing subsidy from public sources, which also help shape both supply and demand. While we do not pursue these tangents, they constitute a part of the complexity in trying to find some order in the fast-changing area of development.

The Nature of Housing and of Living with Assistance

The continuing proliferation of forms of service is an example of both human ingenuity and rising expectations about continuity in normal life with disability and old age. For centuries the extended family and immediate neighbors constituted the major resource for helping the disabled to live at home. Living with family was the most flexible and preferred arrangement; the few other options included group shelters such as hospices and poorhouses and later congregate housing facilities. As early as 1940, it was predicted that Social Security would in time set off a powerful movement away from institutional to private residential life for the aged and disabled but the variety of forms the shift generated was not anticipated (Morris 1961). The recent emergence of so many varieties of personal care services available in connection with residential facilities has surely expanded consumer and patient choices but has also involved constant change as each new form evolved and as both technology and expectations became more complex.

A quite incomplete count of institutional arrangements can begin with 41,483 licensed residential, 8,000 assisted living facilities (Blanchette, AARP), and 700 continuing care retirement communities with an estimated 100,000 to 200,000 residents and with an estimated 15–20 percent annual growth rate in the 1980s (Cohen, Kumar, and McGuire 1991). The assisted living movement began to pick up steam in 1960 and the retirement communities began after 1950.

A Diversity of Examples: What Assisted Living Consists Of

There has been no systematic study of all the variations of service arrangements in what we call the living-at-home service area, but valuable analyses have been made of various components. Drawing on these, we will try to assess the boundaries for a home-care service. AARP has published a useful summary of what assisted living is like in reality, which we also used. This summary is based on information provided by administrators for 63 assisted-living programs in 21 states as well as interviews with major developers, 50 other key informants including professional and consumer groups plus a more intensive look at assisted living in Oregon (Kane).

❃ Median tenant capacity was 56. Facilities ranged in size from 10 to 380 residents.

❃ Forty-one facilities are profitmaking, 22 nonprofit, and half are part of a chain.

❃ Twenty-nine are freestanding facilities built for the purpose or renovated. Nineteen are small sections of housing or congregate care complexes. Eight are owned by nursing homes or homes for the aged. Five are residential parts of a continuing care retirement community.

❃ The average age of residents is 83, and ages range from 65 to 89.

❃ All prefer the fairly independent elderly on admission, but there has been a trend to admit more sick and frail residents. With varying limitations, most will admit or keep residents who use a wheelchair or electric cart, who are incontinent or are mildly or moderately confused. About half will admit or keep those needing transfer help or help with eating. Most admit those using oxygen, catheter, or ostomy. A little over half admit or keep those with behavior problems, while relatively few admit those using a ventilator or who are chairbound.

❃ A few target more affluent patients and most prefer those with few daily living needs.

❃ Several prefer selected ethnic or religious residents, but they seldom exclude others who fit their program.
    The average length of stay was 26 months. While information is not detailed, it appears that most who leave do so because of deteriorating health, moving to a hospital or a nursing home, or they die. In 6 assisted living facilities, however, over 25 percent of those who left returned to independent living.

❃ Median total staff size is 20–21, ranging from 3 to 60.
    There are few medically skilled staff. Thirteen have a staff registered nurse and 15 mention licensed practical nurses; some have on-call arrangements

with a nearby nursing home, but none has a staff physician or medical director. Some residents receive services from home and home health agencies. Staff consists mainly of kitchen and dining room help, maintenance, and activity staff, plus managers and marketers.

❋ Full autonomy is often limited: 44 units do not allow stoves; 22 do not allow microwave ovens; 14 bar refrigerators; and 2 lack private showers, while 13 deny a door key.

❋ Common areas are varied but usually include spacious reception areas, large and small living rooms, recreation room, exercise and entertainment equipment, beauty parlors, laundry rooms, chapels and outdoor areas. In some ways their brochures sound like ads for a vacation resort hotel.

❋ Charges are varied. Seven have a fixed rate but most charge more for especially attractive units or for residents with heavy service needs. The average low rate was $995 a month and the highest $3,800 a month. Half the assisted living facilities receive no public payments for either rent or services.

Blurring the Boundaries: Where Does Assisted Living Fit?

This brief summary makes clear how much the boundaries between homes for the elderly, congregate living, and the private home is beginning to blur. There appears to be a demand for something between a nursing home, which is mainly a medical facility, and a fully independent private home, which the assisted living residence begins to fill. But it has some of the characteristics of a low-skill nursing home, since its residents can have substantial care needs, which were once given in a nursing home. So are assisted living facilities competing with nursing homes? Or are the latter deliberately moving into an upscale medical facility market with more effort to be like home?

At the home-care end of the scale, we cannot help but wonder why many of the residents in an assisted living facility opt for a quasi institution rather than remaining in their own home with extensive at home services delivered. Many assisted living facilities offer some services in addition to shelter and meals, some of which are arranged for by negotiation with a home-care or home-health agency that could deliver the same service to a private home. Is it a matter of cost or convenience for a home-care agency to service groups of patients in one site? Or is it that some (or many) people do not want the responsibilities of maintaining a private home and prefer a quasi hotel—protected—environment because it is seen as both more secure, more protecting in case of need, and offers a more sociable setting for those living alone? Such questions have no clear answer, and this may be a case in which market forces and financing arrangements will determine the changing pattern, not the logical design of health care or social planning. For home-care evolution these questions pose special challenges, discussed later.

Potential Demand for Home-Assistance Services or for Assisted Living

Assisted living in any form is attractive first to those of any age with some serious functional limitation. Chapter 2 has outlined some of the evidence about the population that *might* become interested in alternative options and choices. At least 39 million citizens have conditions that affect their ability to live independently and to go to work or to school; to these can be added the many who begin to think about the future as they age and begin to modify their life patterns. Although only 5 percent of the population overall may be in a nursing home at any one time, it is becoming common for older citizens to think of the 20 percent of elderly alone who can look forward to a nursing home as their energies decrease unless they have made alternate arrangements.

There has been extensive research about the potential for changing these figures without clear evidence about success. The trend in nursing home volume is to concentrate on cases requiring constant or nearly full-time nursing attendance because of the underlying medical and functional condition. Nursing home volume has slowly declined against predicted demand—from the 1972 Congressional Budget Office estimate of 2.2 million residents to an actual 1.5 million in 1985 (CBO 1977).

If we exempt the 5 percent of population in an institution at any one time for cost as well as quality, there remain 95 percent of an at-risk population who may have room to choose among options in this space offered by 11,959 licensed home-health agencies, 41,483 licensed residential care facilities, an unknown number of unlicensed social home-care agencies, 8,000 assisted living facilities, and 700 continuing care residences with an estimated 100,000–200,000 in 1985 and growing 15–20 percent a year. Freestanding day centers, both medical and social, may also be a factor. Taken together they constitute the supply factor to meet either the expressed or hoped for demand. If that demand does not grow the competition may become aggressive for clientele.

The potential demand seems great, but the scope for home-care growth is affected by many aspects of demand. Three population clusters have different potential.

The first cluster includes those who have family for backup support or strong friendship networks as family surrogates. Seventy percent of those over age 55 receive some supportive help, most from unpaid helpers and 91 percent of the much smaller number of disabled receive help. Nearly 74 percent of help is provided only by informal family or other unpaid caregivers. Twenty-one percent receive some combination of paid and unpaid help (Liu, Manton, and Liu 1985). If we think only of those identified by daily living limitations, there are an estimated 5.6 million over age 65 and 3.4 million under 65 at risk, totaling 9 million. Combining all ages, there are estimated to be about 1.9 million disabled already receiving some home care. (National Association for Home Care 1992, cited by Callahan 1996). The gap between 9 million at risk and 1.9 receiving help constitutes a clue to the potential for some service expansion.

The individuals with effective family or close neighbor resources play an important part in a decision to try to maintain one's own home. Such family help as exists is overwhelmingly that of a spouse or adult offspring living nearby. But disentangling evidence about family helping, having a nonhelping family, and family needing supplemental help is difficult. (See Chapter 3 on the role of families.)

The second cluster includes those who lack effective family help and need intermittent but steady medical and nursing attention and may also need daily living care supplementation. Will more or different service patterns increase family help?

The third cluster, having the financial means or private insurance to pay for the added costs of personal care, is available to a small fraction of the potential population, but this fraction influences choices made by service producers who can be attracted to an upscale affluent market first.

The fourth cluster includes those eligible for some tax-subsidized personal care program (mainly SSI, the Veterans Administration, Medicare home health, or Medicaid). Each program imposes its own limit to the scope and type of service for which it pays (e.g., limited to an institution or dependent on concurrent receipt of medical services or otherwise regulated by eligibility for disability benefits or welfare, which frame the window for client choices).

And, finally, the last group, some 28 percent of the aged population, live alone, and almost that percent may have no relevant family ties available. The growth of serial marriages and the drop in the number of children per family erodes some of the base of family support. Offsetting such trends, some family subsets are growing, and the improving health status of the elderly under 80 or 85 is a partial alleviation of the service demand. (See Chapter 3 on the role of families.)

The volume of all home care rises with the prevalence of severe disabilities—another clue to the growth of alternative service patterns as discussed in earlier chapters. For example, those with five disabilities receive an average of 54 hours a week: 10 from a formal agency, 8 from informal visiting care, and 37 from an informal resident helper, usually a spouse (Short and Leon 1990).

Boaz and Hu reported in 1997 the distribution of help-hours when several variables are considered: daily living disabilities, different marital statuses, and different living arrangements. Controlled for need, married persons receive much more help than unmarried ones because of the seldom counted spousal care that supplements any other help. Individuals co-residing with other adults do better than those living alone. The combination of offspring and other adults seems best for unmarried individuals. They conclude that combinations of helpers and living arrangements explain most of the help-hours used by the disabled coping with life at home.

Since so much home care is provided by relatives, it is instructive to note that 63 percent of nursing home residents over 65 have living children, but 81 percent of those living outside of an institution have living children. Nursing home residents are more likely to be widowed or never married; those still living in the community are much more likely to married and a third are widowed (U.S. Department of Health and Human Services 1991, cited by Callahan 1996).

Eighty-one percent of disabled residents with one or two daily living limitations live in the community, whereas 71 percent of those with three limitations are in nursing homes (from Long-Term Care and Nursing Home Surveys 1982, adapted by Leutz, Greenlick, and Capitman 1994). All of this varied information confirms what may be common sense: the more disabled a person is, or is afraid of becoming, the more he or she needs or seeks services or institutional protection. This explains some of the growing interest in assisted living facilities. Untested is whether in-home services could satisfy this need of the more disabled, but the fact that so many do live at home without formal services suggests either that families do not want such help or the services have not yet evolved to meet their wants. Alternatively, home-care agencies have not yet developed their capacities for this population.

The Outlook for Assisted Living

All these numbers suggest that we have perhaps a redundance of refined data but have not had time to reflect on their implications. What do they tell us about a desirable pattern for at-home services and how much should be socially planned or collectively financed and how much left to market choices? Reconciling the flood of numbers is so difficult that there is an impatient tendency to start with an appealing approach and await the results.

This broad excursion through the terrain in which assisted living is finding a place suggests to us that home care, in our earlier narrower definition, will also be affected. All the programs in this "space" are adapting to new conditions. Assisted living seems to have an appeal that suggests that the diversity of human needs, or wants, is not satisfied by the constructs offered by formal service agencies so that new forms are emerging. Assisted living, not yet having a clear shape, has characteristics of some institutions and of some home care.

At least three issues can be suggested:

1. That all service types are elaborating their offerings in a drive to attract more clients-patients. Will they become multipurpose?

2. The theoretical demand for home care, measured by risk populations, seems almost boundless. But will the proliferation of service types mean that all have room to flourish, or is there some as yet ill-defined limit to demand that can lead to more competitiveness?

3. As consumers age, the trade-off between security and home becomes more important. Geographic concentration of services and ready access become important.

Expanding Service Products by Existing Programs— Implications for Home Care

Institutions such as nursing homes, and assisted living facilities to a lesser extent, offer potential clients one advantage over life at home—a concentration in one location of several services that are, presumably, made readily available and can be controlled. For assisted living it is a matter of building on the advantages of geographic concentration of services. From the patient or client point of view, having services concentrated may be comforting, or it may seem to restrict choices arbitrarily, and therefore be less attractive. A family may be secure in the belief that there is staff to maintain surveillance in use of medication and in diet or to look after any unexpected problem or need that may arise. From the agency point of view, it is more efficient to cluster staff and resources with clients-patients in a limited geographic zone or at least one building. Travel from house to house is costly in man hours of labor.

From the point of view of safety, can assisted living facilities demonstrate that their limited staff can actually deliver the promised security of a reasonably accident-free environment or quick access to help. For home care it becomes a matter of reassuring clients or their families that they can handle such worries as well as an assisted living facility with the added advantage of preserving familiar home comforts.

There is not much more than the assurances of any one agency that its services will provide comfort, security, and whatever else is needed as well or better than any other. While much is known about specific client concerns, there is very little research that tries to evaluate what combinations reconcile the desire for choice and freedom with the desire for convenience and safety or security. But many of the types of services discussed here are, each in their own way, trying to adjust and modify their offerings to find the best match they can in the competition for clients or residents.

Nursing homes here and there are adding assisted living components that differ from their basic nursing functions and sometimes offering at-home services when there are waiting lists. Although the tendency is to concentrate on accepting the sickest patients with most service needs, many still have residents with minimum needs. This has been recognized by the number of Medicaid-financed programs using Health Care Finance Administration waivers to offer alternative, less costly service options for nursing home eligible patients. The effects on the institutional role are still being studied.

Hospitals have already added, under an umbrella structure, networks of primary care, outpatient, rehabilitation, and home-care services, all linked and managed from a hospital point of view. Ambulatory surgical centers are provided in order to reduce hospital costs; these shift what were once called convalescent centers for postsurgical care either to the patient's home or to a nursing home, and now perhaps to an assisted living facility. Most of these changes still bring patients to the facility, not the reverse, but they may make services geographically more dispersed—less in the center city and more into several suburbs.

Homes for the aged have for years been adding independent retirement apartment house options with services linked to the home. Their national association has added "services" to their title and some are trying out various day-care or home-care services in tandem with their facility-based program.

Continuing care retirement communities combine housing, food service, property maintenance, socialization, nursing care, and personal assistance under one management and usually at one site. They are still growing. If the Kane survey is accurate, the assisted living label already embraces bits of each of the above. Some offer only housing, leaving all services for the resident to secure; some offer limited personal care, or contract meal and cleaning; others arrange through management to import health and social services.

What distinguishes all these tendencies from home care as we have used the term is that the personal and social services and some of the health services of long-term care can be treated separately. They can be unbundled from the housing component and repackaged differently and delivered in more compact geographic areas. The new package is managed by a basic nonprofit or for-profit corporate entity.

The impetus for these shifts begins with concern over high costs but is more likely to result in shifting costs along the continuum of services and perhaps to the ultimate consumer. One evidence of this shifting may be found in the growing concern that, under Medicare, home-health care services and costs are increasing at an unprecedented rate (Bishop and Skwara 1993, cited by Callahan 1996) while the rate of increase (not total cost) in hospital and nursing home spending seems to have slowed down.

The Dilemma of Consumers Searching for Safety Plus Home

If this very preliminary analysis holds up, the home-care field faces a challenge. Its major justification has been that 75–85 percent of citizens, when polled, prefer to remain in their own homes when ill. But only a minority make use of available services. The field developed its own highly fractionated system of separate agencies. A major division persists between home-health agencies (mainly nursing) and social home-care agencies. The former offer mainly nursing care but some have added personal care functions for the chronic sick as well as contracting for such services for their patients. Social home-care agencies have problems in accepting clients severely limited in daily living abilities. A comprehensive agency could include all of the following, but most are very limited, offering services reflecting their histories: personal assistants, nurses aides, housekeepers, chore and home maintenance, shopping, transportation, personal counseling, and so on.

The result is a dense network of relatively small agencies with varying mechanisms to coordinate their work. This pattern of traditional service has the virtue of flexibility (with complexity) to meet the infinite variety of wants. But the system lacks geographic concentration in the use of resources. One agency may try to rationalize the movement of its personnel to be efficient, but in the aggregate the services lack much concentration except through the cumbersome mechanism of cross referrals.

At the same time, some home-care agencies have begun to contract their services to residents living in some kind of group managed housing, either arranged by the housing manager or with individual residents. Assisted living seems to be a natural venue. The programs we have touched on offer, in some form, freedom from the complexity. They can combine housing with maintenance included plus a management company to which a resident can turn to secure some combination of other health and social services, depending on the contract.

The consumer with more resources can buy freedom from many worries and still maintain control over a personal residence.

Can the traditional care agency system compete? We suggest that the market is not unlimited for them. We think they now need to confront the fragmentation, dispersion of resources, and complexity of their service pattern as affected by the competition, which is changing rapidly. Some of the changes to be considered are discussed further in Chapters 11 and 12.

More Questions Than Answers?

First, is it inevitable that nursing or home-health services and the social support services be organized separately because the professional disciplines are so different, although most potential consumers have some combination of health and social needs? If they must be delivered by different professions or ancillary staff, does this mean that their corporate structures must be separate? If yes, can they be brought together under an umbrella management design much as the institutional services (e.g., hospitals and HMOs) are beginning to do through purchase of some services from other "vendors"?

And, second, how can home-care services combine their target audiences to include the traditional individual client living in a detached home or in an apartment complex in any form? Or to include groups of clients clustered in some group housing whose management seeks home-care services for residents—continuing care retirement communities, assisted living facilities, public housing, or private condominium complexes, or managed retirement communities? Or to include newly defined geographic areas with high concentrations of the elderly or disabled of any age, now called naturally occurring retirement communities that may or may not have some civic associations but do not have health or social service structures specifically for its population (Hunt 1987)? These are relatively compact geographic areas with more than 50 percent of the residents over 60 years of age. It is estimated in one survey that 27 percent of the elderly live in such areas (AARP 1990).

Each of these groupings calls for different staffing, resources, and ways of conceptualizing home care as requiring a group as well as an individual approach to consumers or purchasers. If a group approach is taken, staff skill is needed for marketing, for negotiating charges, for organizing delivery which may well differ from what is involved when an agency waits for a client to apply individually or relies on referral and contract funding from a major payer such as Medicaid, which is not receptive to expansive initiatives.

It is not likely that many of these implied approaches can be handled by home-care agencies as now organized, with their narrow range of staff skills, limited capital resources, small scale and limited social funding.

There are numerous subtle choices and market difficulties that call for more attention than home care has been able to give. For example, in trying to reach out to the large potential untapped home-care demand, should they reach out to groups nowhere near ready to think about a change far in their future? Or how will home care present itself to citizens who, as they are already aware of age, are just beginning to think about a less demanding home. Some will be evaluating whether they need, or want to pay for, all the packaged services offered by some options, including assisted living and other competitive services. How much do they want to trade off privacy, autonomy and choice for packaged benefits at a high cost? At least one continuing care residential community already offers a low entry price, with full refund, but makes available only those services for which residents are willing to pay an added fee as they use the service or are ready to contract for in advance, service by service. Is that much different from living in your own home and buying what you need? It may not be, if the facility is able to organize a fully flexible and individually designed package that is both appealing and low cost.

Also the growing capacity to deliver many technologically advanced services in a private home or in nonmedical group settings calls for upgrading staff skills, paying higher salaries, or adding new staff members and an existing staff and board willingness to take responsibilities for more risky conditions. But home care, as a field, not a single agency, has not yet considered whether some geographic concentration is socially and economically desirable to replace the open door for any who call within a large dispersed area. Neither is it able to offer the kind of assurance about security and convenience that the best institutional facilities do, but at a price beyond the average citizen.

Assisted living developers are able to offer a variety of choices but usually only for those who can afford to pay. What would be useful is better analysis of the mixes of services for which potential home-care clients are ready to pay. Can home care offer different packages of services as an ongoing option, much as is the offer from assisted living facilities that require some trade off in privacy and autonomy for convenience. Unfortunately, consumer choice along these lines is muddied by the reality that most need to think about a future contingency, when their physical energies or capacities may be less, whereas their current desire is to retain their autonomy and life style today, while energies are not declining. Planning or marketing for the future is not a well-defined science but may involve a period of trial and error, which involves risk and capital.

To further complicate the choices, there is a tendency, as privately managed health care is widely adopted and tested, for advocates to demand more and more public control over the service offerings of private insurance in order to protect citizens' interests. It is possible that such regulatory efforts may spread to conventional home care. In a time of skepticism about the drag of top-heavy regulation and the counterpart service agency inexperience with market entrepreneurship, it is unclear how proactive and developmental each form of service will choose to be, and in what direction.

Finally, there is a question whether most of the options are available for the more affluent only. Will services begin to divide along class and income lines? Or will the pressure for each service module try to serve all economic classes but with differential charges or with public subsidy in the interest of equal treatment regardless of cost?

On the hopeful and positive side, this analysis suggests that there is not only inevitable change ahead, but ample opportunity exists for creative steps to be taken without waiting for external events to decide them. Public policy in the use of tax funds can push some changes, but there is room to get ahead of the curve of change, albeit with some unfamiliar risks. The hospital and health fields have reshaped themselves, for better or worse, without waiting for public policy; social programs are beginning to do the same. How can home care respond?

CHAPTER 10　❈　*Toward Improved Financing*

$\mathcal{F}$ORMAL LONG-TERM care services are driven as much by the availability of financing as they are by consumer need for personal assistance. For the 20 percent of personal assistance that is provided by formal sources, third-party financing plays a major role in determining whether care is provided at home or in an institution, the degree to which personal assistance is subordinated to health care, and whether services are long term or temporary. The growth of home- and community-based services in the past twenty-five years has been influenced greatly by the availability of third-party financing. When extensive personal assistance services are provided for long periods of time by paid workers, the costs are substantial. For consumers, the costs are often catastrophic. For that reason, financing issues are central to the future of home care. To illustrate, in 1995, nursing home care cost an average $39,000 a year, or $107 per day, and the rates are significantly higher in some areas. In 1993, federal and state Medicaid spending on institutional care alone was $36.3 billion.

Long-term care financing involves many layers of complexity that reflect conflicting values, historical developments, fragmented government, shortsighted national policies, and special interest politics. As a result, the current system is unnecessarily expensive, inefficient, and not always operating in the best interests of those on whose behalf large amounts of tax dollars are being spent. The fact that the current system costs so much, combined with the public's expressed desire to reduce government spending, presents a window of opportunity to reform and reshape the long-term care system and make it more suitable for the economic and demographic realities facing the nation.

A variety of options have been proposed to strengthen or improve long-term care financing, but all of them have serious limitations. In this chapter we will spell out the qualities we look for in evaluating financing mechanisms, describe existing financing mechanisms, review proposals for improved financing, and propose some directions for the future.

Home-Care Financing

Although most long-term care recipients live outside of institutional settings, the bulk of cash payments for long-term care is for the minority who reside in nursing homes and other institutions. Average payments for persons living in institutions tend to be much higher than payments for those living independently because institutional care implies nearly total reliance upon formal or paid help. For the functionally disabled who live at home paid help tends to supplement self-care and informal personal assistance. Proposals for financing long-term care tend to focus on those who must pay for the high costs associated with institutional care. Because the bills for noninstitutional care tend to be much lower, they are sometimes entirely overlooked in long-term care financing proposals. If the first emphasis in such financing is to cover institutional costs, an inadvertent consequence may be to lead some to seek care in an institution to take advantage of the availability of financing. We will emphasize financing of noninstitutional home care as a way of correcting for the tendency to give it only secondary attention.

Current Sources of Financing

Home- and community-based long-term care is currently financed by a combination of public and private sources. Public third-party payers include Medicare, Medicaid, Older Americans Act, Veterans Administration, Social Services Block Grant programs, and community organizations, such as local chapters of the American Cancer Society, the Alzheimer's Association, and the National Easter Seal Society.

Private third-party payers include commercial health insurance companies, Medigap insurance, long-term care insurance, managed-care organizations, and workers' compensation.

We will review the major sources of financing and the opportunities and limitations they present in relation to personal care services.

MEDICARE

Enacted in 1965 as Title XVIII of the Social Security Act, Medicare is the nation's health insurance program for nearly 39 million aged and disabled persons. Virtually everyone over 65 is insured under Medicare, as well as 5 million disabled persons who are eligible for Social Security Disability benefits. Since the program was established, the Medicare population has doubled, and it is estimated to grow to 55 million in the next twenty years. For 1997, it is estimated the cost of Medicare benefits will amount to $208 billion.

Medicare consists of two parts: Hospital Insurance (Part A), financed mainly by a 1.45 percent payroll tax on earnings paid by employees and employers, and Medical Insurance (Part B), which is financed by a combination of beneficiary payments ($43.80 per month in 1997) and general revenues. Hospital Insurance, Part A, accounts for 58 percent of total program spending. It covers inpatient hospital services, skilled nursing facility payments, home health benefits, and hospice care. For each of these services there are conditions, specific limitations, and in some cases a deductible or coinsurance payment. Part B accounts for 30 percent of program costs and pays for physician services, outpatient hospital services, laboratory procedures, and medical equipment. (The remaining 12 percent of Medicare spending is for managed care plans that provide both Part A and Part B services for enrolled participants.)

The public continues to be surprised that Medicare is not designed to be a source of financing for long-term care. For example, Medicare covers the cost of nursing home care only during a period of recovery from acute health problems. Medicare covers nursing home care fully for 20 days and partially for an additional 80 days, but only in conjunction with the provision of certain therapeutic services. After 100 days, Medicare nursing home payments cease (Health Care Financing Administration 1996). In 1991, Medicare financed only 5 percent of nursing home care (Wiener, Illston, and Hanley 1994).

Medicare also finances home health service, and over the years, it has been liberalized substantially. In an earlier period, Medicare financed home health service only during a period of recuperation from an acute health problem that required hospitalization. While benefits are no longer tied to hospitalization, Medicare provides coverage only when therapeutic care can be justified. Depending on the patient's condition, Medicare may pay for skilled nursing; physical, occupational, and speech therapies; medical social work; and medical equipment and supplies. As a result of the settlement of a lawsuit, *Duggan v. Bowen* in 1988, eligibility criteria have been loosened so that those with either part-time *or* intermittent need are eligible now. (Previously, the need for care had to be both part-time *and* intermittent.) Beneficiaries can receive services for a maximum of eight hours per day, seven days a week.

Medicare home health expenditures have expanded enormously—from $100 million in 1970 to $12.3 billion in 1993. The growth was particularly rapid in the years immediately following the *Duggan v. Brown* decision. In each of the years between 1990 and 1992, growth rates in expenditures exceeded 40 percent. In the period between 1989 and 1992, expenditures increased by 210 percent (Mauser and Miller 1994).

The extent to which the expanded Medicare home health expenditures represent personal assistance services is not entirely clear. A recent study by Hijjazi (1997) based upon the 1993 and 1994 Medicare Beneficiary Survey found that a majority of users of home health services received home health aide services (57 percent in 1993 and 67 percent in 1994). In both years, mean home health aide visits averaged 27. These findings suggest that in typical cases, Medicare home health services had not become a source of frequent personal assistance services for indefinite periods.

Medicare home health benefits have expanded to the point that they are now a focal point for cost-control measures. The Balanced Budget legislation of 1997, for example, targeted the program for a 15 percent reduction in expenditures (CQ Weekly 1997). The consequences of these control initiatives are difficult to anticipate. It is clear, however, that the federal government will seek to prevent the Medicare home health program from becoming a source of financing for intensive, open-ended personal assistance services for beneficiaries.

Hospice services are available to individuals who are terminally ill and have a life expectancy of six months or less; there is no requirement for the patient to be homebound or in need of skilled nursing care. A physician's certification is required to qualify an individual for the Medicare Hospice Benefit. The physician also must recertify the individual at the beginning of each six-month benefit period (Frazer 1985).

As generous as these benefits sound, Medicare covers less than half of total health spending of the elderly and is less generous than health plans typically offered by employers. Medicare has relatively high deductibles, no cap on out-of-pocket expenditures, and no outpatient prescription drug coverage. Beneficiaries spend on average $2,605 out-of-pocket for health services and premiums. Two-thirds of all Medicare beneficiaries have either Medigap (supplemental) insurance or some type of retiree health insurance from an employer. The Medicare premiums, deductibles, and coinsurance for very poor elderly are often paid by their state Medicaid agency.

MEDICAID

Enacted in 1965 as Title XIX of the Social Security Act, Medicaid is a federal-state health care program for public welfare recipients (aged, blind, disabled, and families with dependent children) and other categorically needy persons whose medical costs are so great they would be on welfare if they had to pay them. Medicaid is a state program in which the federal government agrees to pay at least 50 percent of the costs of care provided eligible recipients. Because it is a state program, limits on income eligibility, the number and type of services provided, and provider payment levels differ from state to state. The federal government pays at least 50 percent of Medicaid costs and the states pay the other 50 percent. In 1995, Medicaid provided health and long-term care for 34.8 million persons at a cost of $157.3 billion, $5.5 billion of which was for administration.

In the years since it was enacted, Medicaid has been stretched to become a catchall for helping states pay the costs of health care for various groups and special interests, such as the medically needy, pregnant women, infants, low-income dually eligible Social Security beneficiaries, and the like. In the absence of suitable insurance, large numbers of middle-class elderly persons have "spent down" their assets in order to become eligible for Medicaid-financed nursing home care.

Over 40 percent of all nursing home care nationally is financed by Medicaid. In 1994, 69 percent of nursing home patients relied on Medicaid to pay at least a portion of their nursing home care on a typical day (American Health Care Association 1995). Although Medicaid is designed to serve poor people, it also finances health care for many middle-class people who deplete their assets. Medicaid includes a spend-down provision that enables those with moderate means to purchase health care services to the point that their remaining income and assets fall below the income eligibility threshold. From that point on, Medicaid covers health care costs. A substantial proportion of nursing home patients establish eligibility for Medicaid financing through the spend-down provision. The incidence of Medicaid spend down depends on the method of calculation (Wiener, Sullivan, and Skaggs 1996). The highest estimate is based upon current residents who were admitted on a private pay basis. In this group, 47 percent eventually spent down to the Medicaid level.

Medicaid funds are also used to pay the "disproportionate share hospital adjustment," an additional payment for hospitals that serve a large volume of low-income patients. There is even a Katie Becket provision, which allows Medicaid coverage to be extended to certain disabled children under 18 who are living at home with their parents but who would be eligible for Medicaid if they resided in a hospital, nursing facility, or intermediate care facility for the mentally retarded.

Some perspective on how far Medicaid has been stretched from its original purpose of paying for health care required by public welfare recipients can be seen from these statistics: In 1988, recipients of Aid to Families with Dependent Children (AFDC) and Supplemental Security Income (SIS) accounted for 72 percent of all Medicaid expenditures; in 1994, public welfare recipients accounted for only 58 percent of the costs. Long-term care services accounted for approximately 36 percent of Medicaid expenditures in 1994. Twenty-one percent of the funds went to pay for nursing home care and 6 percent covered home-care expenses for persons living in the community. Another 7 percent financed intermediate-care facilities for the mentally retarded and 2 percent was spent on mental health services.

Medicaid's home health benefits are not restricted to those requiring skilled care (Feder 1991). Further, the Medicaid program has an optional Personal Care provision through which Medicaid may pay for personal assistance services for the disabled. States, therefore, can elect to cover personal assistance services. In addition, since 1981 Congress has authorized states through the 2176 Waiver program to use Medicaid funds to provide home- and community-based long-term care. The aim of the waiver is to encourage community care for populations that would qualify for nursing home care. The waivers can be used for a variety of groups at risk for institutional care including the elderly, the chronically mentally ill, the physically disabled, the retarded, and the nonelderly physically disabled. Federal law permits waiver programs to reach some of those who would not meet Medicaid's usual financial eligibility criteria. Eligibility for waiver services may be extended to include those with incomes up to 300 percent of the poverty level (Feder 1991, 41).

States vary a great deal in the extent to which they have financed long-term care through Medicaid. New York State has made far greater use of Medicaid for long-term care financing than has any other state. In 1986, New York accounted for 60 percent of Medicaid expenditures for home health and personal care combined (Feder 1991, 39). Eighty-six percent of the New York expenditures were for personal care. In New York, Medicaid expenditures per elderly person averaged over $2,500. The emphasis on Medicaid-financed personal care has been particularly strong in New York City. There, a large home attendant program provided an average of over 50 hours of care per week to each client. (More recently, the New York State legislature has prohibited such extensive service authorizations.)

The waiver programs were initially constrained by both state fiscal concerns and a federal requirement that their impact on overall federal long-term care expenditures be neutral. Even though the waivers were expected to attract clients who would never have used nursing home care, they were required to have a neutral effect on overall state long-term care expenditures. Subsequently the program was liberalized to require only that those served through the waiver program be eligible for nursing home care and that they be served at a cost below that of nursing home care. Under federal Medicaid rules, coverage of home health services must include part-time nursing, home-care aide services, and medical supplies and equipment. At the state's option, Medicaid also may cover audiology; physical, occupational, and speech therapies; and medical social services. Hospice is a Medicaid-covered benefit in 38 states. The Medicaid hospice benefit covers the same range of services that Medicare does.

OLDER AMERICANS ACT

Passed by Congress in 1965, the Older Americans Act provides federal funds to support a network of state and local offices of aging. The funds can be used for state and local social service programs that enable frail and disabled older individuals to remain living independently in their communities. For example, in some areas there may be funding available to cover home-care aides, personal care, chore, escort, meal delivery, and shopping services for individuals with the greatest social and financial need who are 60 years of age and older. Increasingly, individuals who can afford to pay for some of these services are being asked to contribute in proportion to their income.

DEPARTMENT OF VETERANS AFFAIRS

Veterans who are at least 50 percent disabled due to a service-related condition are eligible for home health-care coverage provided by the U.S. Department of Veterans Affairs. A physician must authorize these services, which must be delivered through the VA's network of hospital-based home-care units. The VA does not cover nonmedical services provided by home-care agencies.

SOCIAL SERVICES BLOCK GRANT PROGRAMS

In 1975 a federal social services program that provided matching money for state social service expenditures was converted to a block grant program that did not require state matching. States enjoyed substantial freedom in defining the services to be financed and the populations to benefit. Some used the funds largely for child-care programs; others used a portion of the funds to finance home-care services for the elderly. California is a large state that drew extensively upon its block grant funds to finance home care for the elderly. A few states have developed substantial home-care programs for the elderly financed through state funds. In 1986, expenditures for home- and community-based care totaled over $100 per elderly person in seven jurisdictions. In two of them, Alaska and Massachusetts, state funds were the major source of financing. In New York, Maine, and the District of Columbia, Medicaid was the source of a majority of the financing. In California, the major funding came from the Social Service Block Grant. In Washington State, the funding was obtained more evenly from Medicaid, the block grant, and state funds (Lipson and Donohoe 1988, cited in Feder 1991, 37).

Private Third-Party Payers

Commercial health insurance policies typically cover some home-care services for acute needs, but benefits for long-term services vary from plan to plan. Commercial insurers, including Blue Cross and Blue Shield and others, generally pay for skilled professional home-care services with a cost-sharing provision. Such policies occasionally cover personal-care services. Most commercial and private insurance plans will cover comprehensive hospice services, including nursing, social work, therapies, personal care, medications, and medical supplies and equipment. Cost-sharing varies with individual policies but often is not required.

Individuals sometimes find it necessary to purchase Medigap insurance or long-term care insurance policies, for additional home-care coverage. Medigap insurance is designed to bridge some of the gaps in Medicare coverage. Some Medigap policies offer at-home recovery benefits, which pay for some personal care services when the policyholder is receiving Medicare-covered skilled home health services. The policyholder's physician must order this personal care in conjunction with the skilled services. Home-care coverage in Medigap policies is not designed to cover extended long-term care. This type of coverage is most helpful to individuals recovering from acute illness, injuries, or surgery.

Initially, the exclusive aim of long-term care insurance was to protect individuals from the catastrophic expense of a lengthy stay in a nursing home. But as consumer preference for home care has increased and home-care services have become better established, many private long-term care insurance policies have expanded their coverage to address needs of community-residing beneficiaries. Of particular interest for this discussion are policies that emphasize personal assistance rather than home health services. Benefits of personal assistance components of long-term care policies vary on several important dimensions: the form of benefits, the nature and duration of benefits, the conditions that trigger eligibility, and co-payment requirements.

Benefits are provided in two fundamentally different ways: indemnity and service reimbursement. In the case of indemnity policies, beneficiaries receive cash payments that can be used at their discretion. In contrast, service reimbursement policies cover all or a portion of certain approved services. These services may include homemaker, chore, out-of-home day care, out-of-home respite, personal response system, and home-delivered meals. Less likely to be covered are home and property maintenance. Some policies now provide coverage for assisted living.

Because private financing is of major importance for the future of home care, we summarize the findings of several studies of out-of-pocket payments for home care. Stum, Bauer, and Delaney (1996) examined out-of-pocket home-care expenditures for a sample from the 1984 National Long-Term Care Survey. They found mean monthly expenditures of $173 for assistance with any Activity of Daily Living (ADL) task, Instrumental Activity of Daily Living (IADL) task, or nursing service. The distribution was highly skewed. The median expenditure was only $32. Only 10 percent reported paying more than $496 per month. A multiple regression analysis found that assets but not income were related to out-of-pocket expenditures. In a study of 182 family caregivers of persons with dementia, Collins and Stommel (1991) also found that out-of-pocket expenditures varied greatly. They found average monthly expenditures of $383 for services that included physician visits, short-term nursing home stays, medications, and home equipment. Ten percent of the families incurred average monthly expenses above $1,000. Collins and Stommel were largely unsuccessful in explaining the variation in expenditures. In a recent national telephone survey of caregivers 18 years of age and older, the National Alliance for Caregiving and AARP (1997) were able to elicit out-of-pocket expenditure reports from 41 percent of their sample. These respondents reported typical expenditures of $171 per month. Families USA (1994) reports an analysis based upon the National Medical Expenditure Survey that examined spending for a range of health and personal assistance services that included nursing, physical therapists, home health aides, homemakers, doctors, and social workers. In 1993 in instances in which out-of-pocket payments supplemented public payments for long-term care at home, monthly payments averaged $151. One-third received paid care that was entirely out of pocket. For this group monthly payments averaged $314. For those whose paid care was entirely out-of-pocket, the average monthly expenditure was $351 when their income was at least 200 percent of the federal poverty level and $410 when they had three or more ADL deficits.

No doubt the out-of-pocket expenditures reported in these studies are burdensome for many consumers. The monthly money amounts involved, however, are much lower than the amounts involved in financing nursing home care. Consumers are spending more for nursing home care than they are on home care. Also noteworthy is the fact that when public payers are involved with home-care financing, expenditures are much higher than when the care is financed entirely by out-of-pocket payers. When public payers were involved, the average monthly spending was $840; when the cost was covered entirely by consumer, the average monthly spending was $314. Although this comparison does not control for the complexity of the conditions involved, it suggests that consumers are less willing to spend for home care than is the public sector.

For both indemnity and service reimbursement policies, receipt of benefits is triggered by an assessment carried out by an agent of the insurance company. Typically, some number of ADL limitations must be present to establish eligibility for benefits. In some cases, cognitive deficits also trigger benefits. In the case of service reimbursement policies, insurance companies may employ case managers to develop service plans. Reimbursement, then, is limited to services that are included in the plan.

From the perspective of a consumer purchasing long-term care insurance, the relative strength of institutional and noninstitutional components is a major consideration. Our emphasis is on the strength of noninstitutional components. Provisions for community care are stronger when eligibility for benefits is more readily triggered, when the dollar amount of indemnities is greater, when more varied and more frequent services are covered, when benefits are of longer duration, and when waiting periods and co-payments are minimized. Consumers should expect to pay more for policies that offer stronger benefits.

Some companies now offer stand-alone home-care policies. Others sell home-care coverage only as a supplement to nursing home coverage. Holding other factors constant, policies that cover home care alone are less expensive than comprehensive long-term care policies. Stand-alone home-care policies pose a risk for consumers who must balance the lower premiums against the possibility they may eventually need institutional care in spite of their access to home care.

Managed care organizations and other group health plans sometimes include coverage for home-care services. Those contracting with Medicare must provide the full range of Medicare-covered home health services available in a particular geographic area. Medicare beneficiaries who are enrolled with a managed care organization may elect their hospice benefit from the hospice of their choice. These organizations only pay for services that are preapproved.

On a cost-shared basis, the Civilian Health and Medical Program of the Uniformed Services (CHAMPUS) covers skilled nursing care and other professional medical home-care services for dependents of active military personnel and military retirees and their dependents and survivors. CHAMPUS offers a comprehensive hospice benefit to its terminally ill beneficiaries, which covers nursing, social work and counseling services, therapies, personal care, medications, and medical supplies and equipment.

Any individual requiring medically necessary home-care services as a result of injury on the job is eligible to receive coverage through workers' compensation.

Adequacy of Current Financing

The prospect of financing long-term nursing home care is a major challenge for most older people. In 1993, the average annual cost of nursing home care exceeded $38,000 (Wiener, Sullivan, and Skaggs 1996). In 1993, 36 percent of nursing home admissions spent more than 40 percent of their income and assets on care (Wiener, Illston, and Hanley 1994, 41). In 1993, more than a quarter of nursing home admissions spent more that $20,000 out of pocket for nursing home care. Of those who enter nursing homes, 55 percent will experience at least one year of care before they die; 21 percent will have lifetime use of five years or more (Kemper and Murtaugh 1991, 595). Approximately 13 percent of the aged households (couples or unmarried individuals) have incomes over $40,000 per year (Social Security Administration 1996). In short, only a small minority of the elderly can afford to pay for nursing home care themselves on a sustained basis. Wiener and colleagues (1994) conclude that less than one-tenth of the elderly can afford to pay for nursing home care for a year solely on the basis of income. Among those who cannot finance nursing home care on the basis of income, some are able to do so by drawing upon assets. Some of them deplete their assets and draw upon Medicaid to finance their nursing home care.

For the public sector, the growing cost of Medicaid-financed nursing home care is a major challenge. Medicaid expenditures for nursing home care have grown rapidly and are expected to continue to grow rapidly. The Brookings-ICF long-term care financing model projects that the 1993 Medicaid nursing home expenditures of $22.4 billion will grow to $35.4 billion by 2008. Further, Medicare's share is expected to grow from $4.3 billion to $7.6 billion. For the public sector, then, there is major reason to slow the rate of growth in costs of nursing home care.

Home-care expenditures are also expected to grow substantially. According to the Brookings-ICF model, home-care expenditures will increase from $21 billion to $40 billion between 1993 and 2018 (Wiener, Illston, and Hanley 1994, 4). The expectation is that combined Medicaid and Medicare expenditures will increase from $13 billion to $24 billion during that period. As indicated above, the rapid growth of expenditures for the Medicare home health program has alarmed policy makers and led to initiatives to reduce expenditures.

Consumer expenditures for home care have received relatively little attention. The data that are available require careful interpretation. On the basis of the 1989 National Long-Term Care Survey, Burwell and Jackson (1993) reported that 60 percent of consumers who used formal home-care services financed all of the home care themselves. Wiener, Illston, and Hanley (1994), on the other hand, found that consumer expenditures for home care are much lower than those of third-party financing for home care. For 1993, they reported that aggregate consumer expenditures for home care were $5.5 billion compared to $15.2 billion from Medicare, Medicaid, and other sources.

The data suggest that in the instances in which consumers pay for all of the formal home care they receive, their total expenditures are modest. When home care involves third-party financing, the expenditures tend to be much higher. Through an analysis of 1984 National Long-Term Care Survey, Stum, Bauer, and Delaney (1996) found that mean monthly expenditures were $173 for assistance with any ADL tasks, IADL tasks, or nursing service. The distribution was highly skewed. The median expenditure was only $32. Only 10 percent reported paying more than $496 per month. A multiple regression analysis revealed that assets but not income were related to out-of-pocket expenditures. In a study of family caregivers of persons with dementia, Collins and Stommel (1991) also found that out-of-pocket expenditures varied greatly. They found average monthly expenditures of $383 for services that included physician visits, short-term nursing home stays, medications, and home equipment. Ten percent of the families incurred average monthly expenses above $1,000. Collins and Stommel were largely unsuccessful in explaining the variation in expenditures. In a recent national telephone survey of caregivers 18 years of age and older, the National Alliance for Caregiving and AARP (1997) were able to elicit out-of-pocket expenditure reports from 41 percent of their sample. These respondents reported typical expenditures of $171 per month. Families USA (1994) reports an analysis based upon the National Medical Expenditure Survey that examined spending for a range of health and personal assistance services that included nursing, physical therapists, home health aides, homemakers, doctors, and social workers. In 1993, in instances in which out-of-pocket payments supplemented public payments for long-term care at home, monthly payments averaged $151. One-third received paid care that was entirely out of pocket. For this group monthly payments averaged $314. For those whose paid care was entirely out-of-pocket, the average monthly expenditure was $351 when their income was at least 200 percent of the federal poverty level and $410 when they had three or more ADL deficits.

No doubt the out-of-pocket expenditures for home care reported in these studies are burdensome for many consumers. The monthly money amounts involved, however, are much lower than the amounts involved in financing nursing home care. Wiener, Illston, and Hanley (1994) reported that the aggregate consumer out-of-pocket expenditures of $5.5 billion for home care were much lower than the $28 billion spent by consumers through cash income and assets for institutional care. Also noteworthy is the fact that when public payers are involved with home-care financing, expenditures are much higher than when the care is financed entirely by out-of-pocket payers (Families USA 1994). When public payers were involved, the average monthly spending was $840; when the cost was covered entirely by consumer, the average monthly spending was $314. Although this comparison does not control for the complexity of the conditions involved, it suggests that consumers are less willing to spend for home care than is the public sector.

The relatively modest consumer expenditures for home care lend themselves to varied interpretation. One possibility is that consumer out-of-pocket expenditures have been substantially underreported. If consumers purchase goods and services from varied sources to support home care, they may not keep complete records on their expenditures and, hence, may tend to underreport their actual spending. Assuming, however, that the data are valid, consumers may spend modestly because they are able to purchase services more efficiently than can third parties. A direct comparison of consumer out-of-pocket expenditures for home care with consumer expenditures for nursing home care may not be appropriate since nursing home costs include room and board. Another possibility for explaining the differences between out-of-pocket and third-party expenditures for home care is that some consumers may be skeptical about the value received from formal home-care services. Some consumers may accept formal services when they are paid for by a third party but not when they have to pay for the services themselves. The possibility that many potential consumers are skeptical about the value of formal home-care service prices when they themselves have to pay deserves careful consideration.

Proposals to Strengthen Long-Term Care Financing

A good deal of systematic analysis has been conducted in recent years of options for strengthening long-term care financing. The most thorough and sustained work has been done by a team at the Brookings Institution headed initially by

Alice Rivlin and subsequently by Joshua Wiener. The Brookings effort led to two important books, *Caring for the Disabled Elderly: Who Will Pay?* (Rivlin and Wiener 1988) and *Sharing the Burden: Strategies for Public and Private Long-Term Care Insurance* (Wiener, Illston, and Hanley 1994). The Commonwealth Fund Commission on Elderly People Living Alone also carried out a significant initiative on home care for the elderly. A team headed by Diana Rowland published its own substantial volume on long-term care financing with special emphasis on home care (Rowland and Lyons 1991). In addition, a substantial literature has been developing on specific long-term care financing options. Our aim here is to provide an overview of the options and offer our own perspectives on the dilemmas embedded in the financing issues.

Private Insurance

Increasingly, functional disability is seen as a risk that lends itself to coverage through private insurance. An insurance approach is premised on the idea that the risk of experiencing the insured event is relatively low, but for those who experience the event the costs are high. Insurance spreads the risk; a large number of people pay relatively modest premiums with the expectation that they will receive substantial benefits if they experience the insured event. Insurance is widely developed in the private sector. Life, housing, automobiles, health, personal liability, professional liability are among the risks that are now routinely protected through private insurance. Some insurance companies are now persuaded that functional disability is a sufficiently verifiable condition so that it can be used to establish eligibility for nursing home care. Further, insurance companies have also recognized that some long-term care services are sufficiently defined so that they can specify a set of services that can be reimbursed through insurance. A number of companies now market long-term care insurance on an individual and group policy basis. A basic challenge in selling private long-term care insurance stems from the fact that risk of needing long-term care is associated with age. If consumers begin their long-term care insurance early in life, the cost of premiums is relatively modest; however, if consumers purchase policies late in life, the cost of premiums is very high. Wiener, Illston, and Hanley (1994) report that in 1991, the annual premium for individual long-term care policies with inflation protection was $2,500 at age 65; at age 79 the annual rate was $7,700.

To date it has been very difficult for insurance companies to sell policies to middle-aged people. Some of their reluctance to purchase long-term care insurance stems from their underestimation of the likelihood that they will require long-term care services. A recent analysis based upon the Health and Retirement Survey, for example, Salmons (1996) found that, within a sample consisting primarily of people in their fifties, respondents' expectations that they would need nursing home care were 50 percent of their actual risk. The actual risk that persons who turned 65 in 1990 will enter nursing homes before they die is estimated at 43 percent (Kemper and Murtaugh 1991). In the Health and Retirement Survey only 20 percent of the respondents estimated that they had a 50 percent chance or greater of needing long-term care in a nursing home in the future.

A key to the affordability and premium/payout efficiency of long-term care insurance is the successful marketing of group policies. When policies are sold on a group basis, they can be offered at a much more attractive rate than when they are sold individually. Policies are best sold through employee groups. Unfortunately, employers are reluctant to add long-term care insurance to employee benefit packages. Interest in long-term care insurance has risen in a period in which employers are reluctant to add fringe benefits of any kind. Dramatic increases in the costs of employer contributions to health insurance have made it difficult for employers to sustain current benefit packages.

In 1997 through the Health Insurance Portability Act, the federal government provided a tax incentive for purchasing private long-term care insurance. The bill makes it possible under some circumstances for consumers to deduct premiums for long-term care insurance from their federal income tax bills. This tax incentive is likely to be particularly significant for the middle income group that is not eligible for means-tested programs.

Questions about the insurability of long-term care remain. Insurers have reason to be concerned about adverse selection, that is, the tendency for those who are more likely to need service to purchase policies. If benefit claims prove to be much higher than anticipated, insurers may have great difficulty in meeting their obligations. Large companies that sell many insurance products could absorb substantial losses on a single product such as long-term care insurance, but the experience would either lead them to increase rates substantially, weaken their coverage, or perhaps even phase out their long-term care policies.

Also uncertain are the implications of insurance coverage for demand of more attractive long-term care services. Consumers tend to be highly reluctant to move to nursing homes even if cost is not an issue. Certain home-care services might be highly attractive, however, to policyholders. Even if functional disability criteria are used to establish eligibility for long-term care benefits, the attractiveness of certain home-care benefits might result in claims that are substantially greater than anticipated.

Uncertainties about what the policies might buy for them when they claim benefits are a serious concern for consumers who purchase long-term care insurance policies at relatively early ages. Boyd (1990) points out that in 30–40 years long-term care services may be very different from what they are now. If so, consumers may be unpleasantly surprised when they seek benefits. Consumers who purchased policies ten years ago, for example, could not have anticipated the rapid growth of assisted living facilities. Consequently, they would not have sought policies that would provide some coverage for costs of assisted living. If filing claims today, these policyholders have no assurance that their policies will provide any coverage for assisted living.

Some insurance companies are modifying their policies to reflect the growing diversity of long-term care services. Policies currently being offered by several insurance companies illustrate the possibilities for coverage of more diverse services. TIAA offers long-term care policies that not only cover nursing home care but also assisted living, home health, personal assistance at home, adult day care, home modification and case management. The Fortis Long-Term Security Home Care plan includes coverage of home health, adult day care, respite care, and personal assistance. A particularly interesting provision permits personal assistance to be provided by a family member who is certified by a home health agency. CNL offers a long-term care insurance plan that includes nursing home care, assisted living, personal assistance, and adult day care. Finally, Travelers Life Insurance Company covers a smaller set of home health services: nursing, therapy, and personal assistance.

Inflation is also a serious concern for those purchasing private insurance. If the upper limits of benefits are defined in dollars, policyholders may find that benefits claimed twenty to thirty years in the future may purchase far less than anticipated. Better insurance policies now include inflation adjustment features. Inflation protection adds to the cost of policies but should be a high priority for those purchasing policies long before they believe that they will be at serious risk.

Lapsing is a very great concern for private insurance. Insurance companies anticipate that half of their long-term care policyholders will drop their policies within the first five years and approximately 70 percent will drop them within 15 years (Government Accounting Office 1992). The anticipation of high lapse rates makes it possible for insurance companies to offer policies at relatively attractive rates. High lapse rates can also be a source of profits for insurance companies.

From the perspective of concern of population protection for the costs of long-term care, affordability and lapse rates provide reasons for great skepticism about private insurance as a major resource in long-term care financing. Wiener, Illston, and Hanley (1994) summarize a variety of cost studies showing that only 10–20 percent of the elderly can afford long-term care insurance. Currently only 4–5 percent of the elderly have a private long-term care insurance policy (Wiener, Illston, and Hanley 1994). Furthermore, of those who do purchase long-term care insurance, a majority drop their policies before they need long-term care.

Out-of-Pocket Payments

Less attention has been given to those who privately finance home care. Substantial nonmedical home-care services can be purchased for $1,000 a month or $12,000 per year. These, of course, are added to ordinary living expenses. For a significant number of older people, it is possible to find funds from savings and income to cover personal assistance services above and beyond other expenses. The potential for consumer financing of home care through current income depends in part on the scope of the service package, the rates of payment for personal assistance workers and other personnel, household income, and household size. For illustrative purposes, we show the extent to which self-financing of home care may be possible under various conditions in Table 2. Our illustration assumes a person with a combined need for long-term personal assistance and health services. We assume an individual who would benefit from 30 hours a week of personal assistance, 12 hours a week of help from a nursing aide, and 4 hours a week of the services of a registered nurse. We assume that all workers including personal assistants would be paid the federal minimum wage and that the consumer would also cover the cost of the employer contributions to the Social Security and Medicare trust funds. We consider the situation of consumers at three income levels. We also distinguish between consumers who live alone and those who live in a four-person household. We assume that households cover the cost of basic living necessities and a moderate life style before they begin paying for personal assistance and nursing services.

We find that those with incomes of $125,000 are able to afford a full package that includes personal assistance, a nurse aide, and a registered nurse. In the families with $75,000 in income, the individual living alone can afford more than the family of four. In both household sizes, a personal assistant is affordable at an income of $75,000. However, families at this income level cannot afford the full package. The single individual at $75,000 may also be able to purchase the services of both a personal assistant and a nursing aide. At an income level of $35,000, an individual living along is likely to be able to afford the per-

TABLE 2. Estimated Costs and Affordability of Personal Assistance/Home Care

ESTIMATED COSTS

Position	Hours per Week	Hourly Rate	Weekly Cost	Annual Cost
Personal assistant	30	$5.50	$165	$8,580
Nurse aide	12	12.00	144	7,488
Registered nurse	4	25.00	100	5,200
Total			$409	$21,268

ESTIMATED AFFORDABILITY

Family Income	Household Composition	Personal Assistant	Nurse Aide	Registered Nurse
$35,000	3 or more	No	No	No
35,000	Single person	Yes	No	No
75,000	3 or more	Yes	Uncertain	No
75,000	Single person	Yes	Yes	No
125,000	3 or more	Yes	Yes	Yes
125,000	Single person	Yes	Yes	Yes

sonal assistant. However, a household of four with an income level of $35,000 will not be able to purchase any services at all.

These figures illustrate the circumstances that affect the capacity of households to purchase personal assistance and other long-term care services. For those needing less assistance, the capacity to purchase adequate care will extend to lower income households. For those needing more assistance, only higher income households will be able to purchase all the care that is needed.

A mechanism that has been proposed to encourage private savings for long-term care costs is a tax-advantaged savings account for long-term care. The savings in these accounts would be tax sheltered. Legislation permitting development of medical savings accounts has received serious congressional attention as an optional alternative to Medicare. In the Medicare context, the proposed savings accounts are controversial because they are expected to be attractive to healthier more affluent people with fewer health care needs. The concern is that such savings accounts would leave Medicare with the older people requiring more expensive care. Further, Medicare would lose an important upper-income constituency. Since there is no universal national public long-term care program, tax-sheltered savings accounts dedicated to long-term care would not pose the same threat and might stimulate some significant savings.

A disadvantage of a strategy that encourages private savings to cover long-term care costs is that it is inefficient in its aggregate use of resources. Much more money is set aside to cover long-term care costs than is ultimately needed. In the aggregate, an insurance strategy is more efficient because the amount set aside approximates the actual total cost (assuming that substantial revenues are not drawn off for administrative costs and profits). On the other hand, more affluent older people need not regard money saved but not spent for long-term care as money wasted. They may gain satisfaction from the anticipation of leaving money to relatives or charities.

An important characteristic of private savings as a payment mechanism for long-term care is that it provides the consumer with complete choice in the manner in which the resources are used and when they are used. The consumer can decide when needs are great enough to justify spending for long-term care services. The consumer can also decide exactly what service to obtain. The consumer need not be limited to the licensed professional service for which some insurance programs might provide reimbursement. Consumers needing guidance in selecting long-term care services, can hire a private case manager to provide help. In practice, this freedom may be a mixed blessing. Some consumers may use their savings unwisely, spending it too rapidly or paying too much for services. Others may be excessively cautious, neglecting their long-term care needs from fear about their ability to meet other needs that never come.

Expanded Medicaid Coverage

Medicaid is already the major source of financing for nursing home care. One option is to acknowledge Medicaid's role in financing long-term care and to extend explicitly Medicaid's role in financing long-term care for middle-income people. An important aspect of that option is to increase Medicaid's financing of home- and community-based services.

A proposal to expand Medicaid's role in financing long-term care runs counter to concerns about the rapid growth of Medicaid and long-term care's significant role in overall Medicaid expenditures. Proposals to acknowledge Medicaid's role in financing long-term care for the middle class also must address concerns about middle-class people who are hiding assets so that they can qualify for Medicaid-financed long-term care services.

A challenge in discussing Medicaid expansion as an option is that each state has its own Medicaid program. An optimistic interpretation is that each state has a program that is suited to its specific needs and that each state would extend its Medicaid program as it saw fit.

A potential advantage in building upon existing Medicaid programs is that they do have a framework for establishing eligibility, mechanisms for regulating providers, and procedures for paying bills. At the same time, Medicaid can be seen as a program that is dominated by concerns about controlling expenditures. Much of its agenda is to restrict the numbers who establish eligibility and to minimize the use of services. Difficulties that applicants experience in establishing financial eligibility for Medicaid are widespread. Applicants must establish positive evidence that they meet the financial eligibility criteria. Often it is difficult for them to do so. In some states, Medicaid's reimbursement rates are so low that many providers refuse to accept Medicaid patients. Further, Medicaid is generally perceived as a program for poor people. Some middle-class people may be reluctant to use Medicaid-financed services because of its stigma as a program for the poor. The counter argument to concerns about the link between Medicaid and poverty is that the addition of a middle-class constituency may benefit all users. A vocal middle class may be effective in insisting on more humane and efficient processing of applications and more adequate payments to providers.

Medicaid's primary mission in financing health care has positive and negative implications. The positive aspect is its ability to encourage continuity between the health care and personal assistance aspects of long-term care. The negative aspect is the potential for imbalance between attention to health care and personal assistance. Medicaid programs, for example, may be reluctant to provide services to those needing personal assistance in the absence of need for professional heath care. When Medicaid reimburses for personal care, it may do so solely upon the basis of income and disability criteria. However, personal care is an optional benefit; states are not required to pay for personal care.

Medicaid's status as a health care financing program has other interesting implications. Medicaid is an individual entitlement to health care. No assumptions are made about family members contributing to care. In Medicaid-financed home-care programs, family willingness to participate in providing care cannot be made a condition for receiving benefits. Medicaid legislation also prohibits the hiring of close relatives as providers. In the case of personal assistance services, relatives can be cost-effective providers. A few states have found a partial way to work around the Medicaid prohibition on paying relatives who provide personal care services by limiting the restriction to immediate family. Expansion of Medicaid as a payment mechanism for home- and community-based long-term care might be accompanied by a reconsideration of the Medicaid policy for reimbursing relatives for providing personal assistance.

PUBLIC-PRIVATE PARTNERSHIPS

Developed and encouraged through a series of demonstration projects financed by the Robert Wood Johnson Foundation, the partnerships bring together private insurance and Medicaid. The partnerships are aimed at middle-income elderly who have assets but are at risk of losing their assets if they require expensive long-term care services. These older people would eventually draw upon Medicaid to finance their nursing home care. The partnership programs allow purchasers of insurance to protect assets up to the amount of the insurance. The insured become eligible for Medicaid-financed long-term care without depleting the assets that have been protected. The greater the face value of the insurance, the greater the assets that are protected. The approach is particularly attractive to older people who wish to protect assets either for a spouse or the beneficiaries of their wills. The partnerships provide the elderly with a legitimate alternative to illegal asset-transfer strategies that are used to establish eligibility for Medicaid-financed nursing home care. Partnership projects have been established in California, Connecticut, Indiana, Iowa, and New York. The New York model is somewhat different from the others. In New York, the elderly must purchase policies that provide three years of coverage for home care or nursing home care with coverage of a minimum of $100 per day for services. In New York, the plan then protects all of the policyholder's assets, not just the amount covered.

Appraisal of the partnerships in part reflects the critics' views of Medicaid as a vehicle for financing long-term care. Those who are concerned that Medicaid financing has negative implications for access to and quality of long-term care tend to be skeptical about the partnerships as a financing strategy (Wiener, Illston, and Hanley 1994). On the other hand, the partnerships can strengthen the stake of the middle class in Medicaid financing for long-term care. Indirectly, the partnerships may provide political support for Medicaid's role in long-term care to the benefit of all who receive Medicaid-financed services.

SOCIAL INSURANCE

Social insurance has been discussed as a means of assuring long-term care financing protection for the disabled of all ages, including children and non-elderly adults. Because of the cost of comprehensive social insurance that would cover both home care and nursing home care, a number of scaled-down versions of social insurance have been proposed. One would cover home care only; another would cover home care and "front-end" nursing home care; and a third would cover home care and "back-end" nursing home care. "Front-end" strategies would extend Medicare coverage at the beginning of nursing home stays; they would not provide additional protection for those requiring long-term nursing home care. "Back-end" policies would provide protection after a major deductible was satisfied. "Back-end" protection might be designed for those requiring more than two years of long-term care. The elderly would be responsible for the first two years either by drawing on income and savings for private insurance.

The Commonwealth Fund Living at Home initiative proposed a social insurance approach that would build upon the Medicare program. The proposal would cover skilled care, rehabilitative services, and various personal assistance services. The plan included 20 percent cost sharing with the Medicaid program covering the cost sharing for the poor. Eligibility would be based upon daily living deficits or severe cognitive deficits. In 1989, the plan was projected to serve 1.6–2.4 million at a net cost of $6.8 to $10.8 billion. (With less restrictive eligibility criteria, the program would have served more people and cost more.)

The Brookings Institution recommendations for improving long-term care financing call for a combination of private and public initiatives. In the private sector they call for initiatives that encourage self-payment on the part of those who can afford to pay. They call for the federal government to play a strong role in consumer education. They also call for the development of more employer-sponsored long-term care policies that would reach the population under 65 years of age. They recommend favorable tax incentives for private long-term care insurance so that contributions and benefits would not be treated as taxable income.

Because of their skepticism about the extent to which private long-term care insurance will be purchased, the Brookings group places primary reliance upon a social insurance model. They propose to cover a range of home- and community-based long-term care services for the severely disabled and the first six months of nursing home care through a universal program open to all regardless of income. Benefits would be restricted to those who met strict functional disability criteria. Consumers would be responsible for 20 percent of the costs of the services. The Brookings team envisioned that the program would be administered by the states and would require that states match federal funds. The program would not operate as an entitlement program. Instead, the program would operate on a fixed budget basis and services would be offered on a funds available basis.

The Brookings group also called for expansion of Medicaid benefits. They proposed that for those with Medicaid coverage, Medicaid would provide the home-care cost sharing in their proposed insurance approach to long-term care financing. For nursing home residents, they proposed an increased personal needs allowance and a higher level of protected assets.

In 1993, the Brookings group estimated that a comprehensive program with Medicaid liberalization and a social insurance approach to both home care and nursing home care would have an incremental cost of $49 billion. The incremental cost of the home-care component alone was estimated at $21 billion (Wiener, Illston, and Hanley 1994, 27). The comprehensive approach would have more than doubled public long-term care expenditures. The home-care component alone would have increased public long-term care expenditures by nearly 50 percent (Wiener, Illston, and Hanley 1994, 27).

Reflecting popular resistance to federal taxes and federal administration of programs, the Brookings group proposed that the program be administered by states, that the states participate in financing, and that the program operate on a fixed budget. State participation in financing would reduce the federal government's responsibility for the costs. The fixed-budget approach is intended to provide protection against the possibility of runaway costs. The proposed administration through states builds upon the fact that many states have experience in administering home-care programs either through state-funded initiatives or through Medicaid waiver programs.

The long-term care provisions in the Clinton health reform proposal emphasized home- and community-based care because of the preference of consumers for home care and the relatively underdeveloped status of noninstitutional long-term care. Like the Pepper Commission, Commonwealth Fund, and Brookings proposals, the Clinton plan called for funding of a variety of home- and community-based care through programs administered by states on a nonentitlement basis.

Like private insurance plans, social insurance requires a procedure for establishing eligibility. All of the recent social insurance proposals rely heavily upon daily living deficits as a basis for establishing eligibility for long-term care. Some would require only one daily living deficit; others would require at least two. Those lacking only in instrumental daily living abilities that are essential to successful functioning outside of institutions would not be eligible. An administrative framework for determining eligibility would be required. The federal government, for example, might contract with private organizations or states to administer eligibility determination.

Financing Social Insurance through Social Security

Yung-Ping Chen has proposed Social Security as a source of financing for a portion of long-term care through social insurance (Chen 1993). Chen envisions three sources of long-term care financing: personal savings, private insurance, and social insurance. Chen proposes a trade-off between Social Security income and a social insurance program for long-term care financing. The proposal calls for drawing off 5 percent of Social Security benefits to finance a universal public long-term care insurance program. Contributions would be mandatory except for low-income older people for whom Social Security is the sole source of retirement income. In 1991, a 5 percent transfer of Social Security cash benefits to a public long-term care financing program would have generated $15 billion or enough to pay for one quarter of all long-term care costs in that year. Chen proposes a gradual approach to the development of a long-term care trust fund. In the first year 1 percent of Social Security benefits would be placed in the trust fund. In subsequent years, the percent set aside would increase by 1 percent until the fifth year when 5 percent would be set aside. Chen estimated that if his plan had been introduced in 1993, the fund would have accumulated almost $60 billion by 1997. Chen proposes that the system be allowed to accumulate assets for several years before it begins to pay benefits. (The Social Security program began in this way.) With this gradual introduction of the program, Social Security beneficiaries would not notice a decrease in their pensions. Instead they would experience a reduced cost of living adjustment. In short, Chen's plan appears to be a relatively painless method of raising a large sum of money to finance a significant portion of long-term care. Although Chen proposes that a public long-term care financing program cover 85 percent of nursing home costs for those staying more than 90 days and less than a year, some or all of the moneys raised could be used for home and community care.

The major question about the feasibility of the Chen long-term care financing plan is political. As Chen points out, support is most likely from the middle-income elderly who have some assets to protect but are not sufficiently affluent to pay for nursing home care. Low-income older people are likely to be indifferent because they expect that Medicaid will be the major source of financing if they need long-term care. Those with very strong financial resources are not likely to anticipate a need for long-term care insurance.

If incorporated into a legislative proposal that received serious congressional consideration, some criticism can be anticipated that focuses on the mandatory nature of the proposal. Some advocates for Social Security beneficiaries might argue that the plan sets a dangerous precedent in setting aside a portion of benefits before they reach beneficiaries. Because the plan calls for drawing off only 5 percent of benefits, the threat to Social Security cash payments would be more symbolic than actual.

Discussion

A social insurance model that would provide universal or near universal coverage for some aspect of long-term care is highly unlikely in the current political climate. Apart from the fact that the dollar cost of a long-term care insurance package would be substantial, social insurance faces other major obstacles. The federal government has fallen into disfavor as a means of addressing domestic problems. Furthermore, the federal government is challenged to sustain existing entitlement programs that primarily benefit the elderly, notably Social Security and Medicare. Social Security costs are attracting attention in part because of the aging of the population. Because people are living longer and the baby-boom generation is aging, the ratio of people of working age to older Social Security beneficiaries will become much less favorable. Because Social Security is primarily financed through current earnings, the burden of financing Social Security will become substantially greater unless the country realizes significant productivity gains. The burden of financing Medicare has increased dramatically because of both the increase in numbers of older people, inflation in health care costs, and the widening scope of health care services. In a climate in which cuts are being proposed in both Medicare and Social Security, it is unrealistic to expect sufficient support for a major new social insurance program focused on long-term care (Meiners 1984).

Even the attractiveness of the Chen Social Security trade-off proposal for financing a public long-term care financing program is not likely to receive serious consideration in this environment. If politicians anticipated that it would be politically feasible to draw off 5 percent of Social Security benefits for another purpose, some might propose an alternate use of such a fund, such as bolstering the Medicare Trust Fund.

If financing were not an overwhelming obstacle to a social insurance approach to financing home care, the proposed federal-state partnership in the administration of the long-term care provisions in the Clinton program would have received more critical scrutiny. The interest in state administration stems more from negative opinions about federal administration than it does from evidence about the effectiveness of states in administration of public home and community-based care programs. State experience with the administration of home-care programs is largely limited to means-tested programs. A program designed to serve the entire disabled population regardless of income could anticipate a far more demanding constituency than do means-tested programs. If a social insurance approach were to attract substantial public support, the public would have to be persuaded that its eligibility criteria were fair and that its administration were efficient and sensitive to clients.

Most feasible in the current environment is more extensive private financing of long-term care. Most of this will be for the growing numbers who can afford to purchase substantial care themselves. Some of the potential for attracting more private money to long-term care is through private insurance. Most constructive will be efforts to encourage consumers to purchase policies long before long-term care services are needed. These policies will be useful only if the pricing and marketing encourages policyholders to keep up their policies until they die or need long-term care (Crown, Capitman, and Leutz 1992).

Long-term care insurance policies need to be structured so that they provide strong protection for personal assistance needs. We are encouraged by recent evidence that some insurance companies are now offering policies with strong personal assistance benefits at attractive prices. Policies should include extensive home- and community-care benefits to complement nursing home benefits. Benefits should be triggered as soon as need for personal assistance is substantial. Both cognitive deficits and multiple daily living needs should be sufficient to trigger eligibility. Indemnity policies should be encouraged because they provide greater consumer choice. Dollar for dollar, an informed consumer can usually obtain more needed assistance from cash than a service benefit. Policies that offer service benefits should cover the widest possible range of service alternatives. Beneficiaries and their families should play a strong role in the service planning process. Some deductibles and co-payments are desirable as a way of keeping down the cost of policies. Policies should be structured so that they supplement what consumers can be expected to cover through out-of-pocket payments. For the most part, those who can afford long-term care insurance can also afford some out-of-pocket payments for personal assistance at home.

Private long-term care insurance with strong personal assistance benefits will be a feasible option for a much larger portion of the population if premiums can be reduced. Very recent experiences of the Robert Johnson Foundation Public-Private Partnership demonstration in California suggest the potential for more affordable policies. California has legislated new long-term care insurance standards for group policies for retired state employees. Insurers offering policies to members of the California Public Employees Retirement System must include personal assistance benefits that are triggered by daily living deficiencies, cognitive impairment, or complex but stable medical conditions. A number of insurance companies are offering policies to members of the retirement system at $1,200 per year to those who are 60 years of age, at $2,200 per year to those 70 years of age, and $4,300 per year to those who are 80 years of age. The policies provide 3 years of benefits, $120 per day for nursing home care and $60 per day for home care (Clark 1996). Presumably the opportunity to market policies to members of a group helps to account for the modest cost.

Tax incentives like the one included in the 1997 Health Insurance Portability Act can also provide useful encouragement to middle-income people to purchase long-term care insurance. Particularly useful from a federal policy perspective are tax incentives for private long-term care insurance for the middle-income people for whom insurance benefits will prevent spending down to the level at which they would become covered through safety-net programs.

Home equity is another potential source of private financing for long-term care. Through direct communication with the authors, Yung-Ping Chen has recommended use of reverse mortgages to finance long-term care insurance for older people with substantial equity in their homes. The potential for older people to use reverse mortgages to supplement their incomes has previously received attention (Scholen and Chen 1980). The specific suggestion to use home equity to finance long-term care insurance is new. Chen recommends the use of this resource to finance insurance rather than services because, as indicated above, insurance spreads risks.

If widely available, these premium costs could make insurance with personal assistance protection affordable to much of the population. Expanded long-term care coverage would provide an opportunity for personal assistance providers to develop a larger and more stable base for financing than now exists.

Also to be encouraged is private savings for long-term care as part of late-life financial planning. Although a savings strategy is less efficient than an insurance strategy, it may appeal to many older people if it is coupled with an inheritance strategy. People may set aside money if they anticipate that it will either be used to meet long-term care needs or be passed along to surviving relatives.

More extensive expenditures from current income and savings should also be encouraged. Older people and their relatives are spending to a far greater extent for nursing home care than they are for home and community-based long-term care. The widely expressed preference for home care suggests that more money should be spent for home care than institutional care. Spending for home- and community-based care can be more efficient than spending for institutional care. For those with limited needs for assistance, home- and community-based care can be focused upon the specific interventions that are needed. Institutionalization requires payment for a very comprehensive service package.

More effective consumer education is needed to assist the elderly and their families to understand when spending for home- and community-based care is in their interest. Consumers must learn when it is in their interest to purchase assistance with tasks that they previously were able to perform independently. Consumers must also learn to reduce their fears about depletion of their savings. As indicated above, some can extend their independent living in the community by judicious use of reverse-equity mortgages. Given the current funding bias in favor of institutional care, some might have to anticipate institutional care if they ran through their own savings. Yet, by spending for home and community care, they may be able to sustain a relatively independent life for a long period of time.

CHAPTER 11 ❄ *Roles for Professionals*

$\mathcal{T}$HE HOME-CARE field consists of a variety of work roles in addition to those directly involved in providing personal assistance. In chapter 4, we discussed homemakers, home health aides, and other who provide assistance to people with self-care deficits in coping with daily living tasks. In this chapter we focus on professionals who contribute to home care in other ways. The home-care field also includes those who are extensively involved in designing, marketing, and administering claims for private long-term care insurance, in providing legal advice in estate planning to families concerned about long-term care costs, financial planners who help people save in anticipation of long-term care costs, architects who design residences to accommodate the disabled, hardware and software engineers who design assistive devices, planners and administrators of assisted living facilities, and program developers and administrators of various community services like home-delivered meals, out-of-home respite services, and specialized transportation that supports home care.

Many occupations are now considered professions. The distinguishing features of professions include a substantial body of knowledge that provides the basis for practice, a formal system of preparation for entry into the field that combines formal education with practical experience, a credentialing method to establish eligibility to practice independently, a set of standards for professional practice, and often an organized means of monitoring performance. Licensing provides designated professional bodies with the force of law to enforce professional standards. Licensing bodies regulate admission to the field and have authority to revoke the right to practice of those who violate standards. A number of the occupations involved in home care are established or emerging professions.

This chapter concentrates on case managers who play a major role in the administration of home-care programs. Some members of established professions, notably nursing and social work, are engaged in case management in home care; however, many case managers are not members of one of these established professions. In this chapter we will report on efforts on the part of case managers in home care to gain recognition as a new profession.

Case Management

The case management role in contemporary home care developed initially within publicly funded programs designed to provide a coordinated set of community-based long-term care services. Within these organizations, the case management role will shift somewhat as these organizations continue to evolve. Some of the more significant developments in case management, however, are likely to take place in privately funded long-term care services.

Both community nursing and social work have played central roles in the evolution of personal assistance services. As employees of either visiting nurse associations or local public health departments, community nurses have long been involved in providing direct services to patients with serious chronic illnesses and disabilities who continue to reside in the community. Traditionally, community nurses have provided assessment, care planning, and advocacy (Williams 1993). Through both family service agencies and public welfare agencies, social case workers have also long provided services to people with disabilities in the community. Traditionally, the assistance provided by case workers has included counseling, advocacy, and arrangement of limited homemaker or housekeeper services.

With the emergence of publicly financed home-care programs in the 1970s, case management emerged as a specialization distinct from case work and community health nursing. The basic responsibilities of contemporary case managers include assessment, recommending services, arranging for services, care monitoring, and reassessment. The contemporary case manager involved in the administration of a publicly funded home-care program is a gatekeeper whose responsibility is to assure that services are authorized only for those who meet explicit eligibility criteria and that spending for services remains within well-defined limits. At the same time the case manager representing a public funding source typically is also expected to be an agent working on behalf of clients.

The challenges experienced by case managers are affected by funding arrangements. Typically public sector programs operate within a fixed budget framework, that is, agencies have a set amount each year that is available for client services. Agencies typically have well-structured guidelines for service authorizations. Customarily, in these programs, case managers are highly constrained in authorizing services because the money amounts available for services are very limited. A major responsibility for case managers in these situations is to search for other formal and informal resources that can be called upon to assist clients. To be effective in rounding out service packages, the case manager must be highly knowledgeable about resources, creative in drawing upon them, persistent in tracking applications for other benefits, and persuasive in encouraging relatives and friends to take on larger responsibilities.

Managed health care provides a newer context for case management in long-term care. In managed care, funding is capitated; that is, agencies receive fixed funding on a per client basis and are responsible for providing comprehensive services. The managed care model has been introduced in home care through programs like PACE and the social health maintenance organizations that link health care and personal assistance (Chapter 8). The provider draws upon a single pool of funds for both health care and personal assistance. The stakes are higher for case managers in the managed care model than in more traditional case management because claims for personal assistance must be reconciled with those for health care and the greater emphasis in managed care in demonstrating a relationship between services and outcomes. In an integrated health and personal assistance program, the case manager must have some expertise in both health care and personal assistance.

Expenditures for case management in publicly funded programs are often significant. In the Massachusetts state-funded home-care program, for example, case management costs average $80 per month per client. Service authorizations are limited to $189 per month. Case management, therefore, represents 30 percent of the cost of client services (Glickman, Caro, and Stocker 1997). Williams (1993) estimates that the cost of case management nationally varies from $49 to $145 per client per month.

The significance of the contribution made by case management in long-term care is in dispute. Some observers regard case management as a fundamental, essential long-term care service. Others are very skeptical about its contribution and tend to view expenditures for case management as wasteful (Callahan 1989). For third-parties who finance services, the assessment and reassessment aspects of case management are essential in controlling costs. At a minimum, case managers serve as gatekeepers who exclude those who fail to meet eligibility criteria. The service planning and service coordination aspects of case management are most readily justified when clients have multiple service needs (Haslanger 1995).

The movement toward greater consumer direction in home-care programs financed through third parties implies a diminished role for traditional case managers (Chapter 5). The consumer-directed model may limit the professional case management role to eligibility determination, periodic reassessment, and occasional advising on strategies for effective use of benefits. It also looks upon traditional, more expansive case management as an expense that competes with funds that may benefit consumers in other ways. If consumers are to seek advice from case managers in organizing and monitoring long-term care, case managers will have to do more to persuade consumers that their advice is worth paying for. In the consumer-directed model, consumers may be interested in purchasing services that help them with the personnel administration responsibilities that go with hiring their own personal assistance workers. The help that they seek, then, is likely to be very specific to their responsibilities as employers in withholding Social Security payments, making workers' compensation insurance payments, and withholding income tax payments.

Private case management in long-term care, which achieved recognition as a distinct specialty in the 1980s, is of growing importance. In recent years increasing numbers of professionals have established their own case-management services on a fee basis to serve clients who are prepared to pay for long-term care services themselves. Characteristically, they are paid by the consumers who employ them. Private case managers offer a menu of traditional case management services. Consumers select the specific services they want. In some cases, consumers seek only an assessment and service recommendations, so they counsel about residential options. In others, consumers seek help in identifying and selecting service providers. Occasionally, private case managers serve as agents of their clients in making hiring arrangements for personal assistance workers. At times, private case managers serve families as well as an individual patient. They monitor services and the well-being of the service recipient on behalf of distant relatives. The client advocacy role is not compromised by the gatekeeping role in more traditional case management (Rosenberg 1995). The private case manager is either a consultant to the consumer or an agent who acts on behalf of the consumer. The case manager must persuade the consumer of the merit of the service. The case manager cannot claim authority as the agent of source of payment for services. The growing number of older people with the capacity to pay for long-term care services themselves offers the potential for substantial growth in private case management. The extent to which that growth will be realized will depend upon the ability of professionals to offer services that consumers find valuable enough to purchase.

Insurance companies offering long-term care insurance increasingly make use of case managers. Some insurance companies employ their own case managers; others contract with private case management organizations for assessments and service planning. (As long as the market for long-term care insurance remains relatively small and policyholders are scattered around the country, it is more economical for insurance companies to contract with private case management organizations where policyholders live on an as-needed basis than to employ their own case managers.) As indicated in Chapter 10, private insurance companies assess policyholders who claim long-term care benefits to determine whether they meet eligibility criteria. Benefits may be either in the form of cash or services. Particularly when policies offer service benefits, case managers representing private insurance companies perform roles very similar to those performed by case managers on behalf of public agencies when they assess service eligibility and develop service plans. Some insurance companies expect the case managers who represent them to provide policyholders with advice about the relative merits of various residential options and service strategies that can support home care.

California has pioneered in the development of long-term care policies for state employees in which private case management is part of the benefit package. California regulations require that case managers be independent of insurance companies to prevent potential conflict of interest that can arise when case managers are employed by insurance companies. (When employed by an insurance company, a case manager may be under pressure to recommend long-term care services that minimize cost to the insurance company—to the detriment of the policyholder.)

The nationwide markets of insurance companies offering long-term care policies have led to the formation of national networks of private case management organizations. The insurance companies use the networks to identify case management organizations that they can draw upon anywhere in the country. One of them, the National Case Management Partnership has introduced a voluntary accreditation process for case management providers. The accreditation process is designed to provide insurance companies and other customers with assurance that certified case management organizations meet minimum quality standards. At present, accreditation is based entirely upon structural characteristics of case management organizations such as qualifications of staff and evidence of procedural guidelines for systematic application of established case management principles (Gruman 1997).

The networks also assist adult offspring who are geographically separated from a parent needing long-term care in identifying local private case managers. Two such networks have been established, the Integrated Services Network and the National Case Management Partnership (Mahoney et al. 1996).

The extent of educational preparation required for case management has been relatively modest. For many case management positions, only a bachelor's degree is required. In some instances only a two-year college degree is required. Supervisors of case managers are often expected to have master's degrees.

A sign of emerging professionalization of case management for home care is the formation of a professional organization, the National Association of Professional Geriatric Care Managers (Mahoney et al. 1996). The organization represents private practitioners and employees of both public and not-for-profit organizations. Further evidence of the professionalization of case management in long-term care is the creation of the National Academy of Certified Care Managers. The academy offers a testing process through which case managers may obtain professional certification.

Future Directions

As the long-term care field matures, case managers will continue to be needed in home- and community-based long-term care programs that are financed through third parties for assessment and service planning purposes. With greater emphasis on client self-direction, however, the traditional case management role in planning and arranging services is likely to diminish or change its function.

The case management role may be most prominent in managed health-care settings for patients with both serious chronic illnesses and long-term disability. The large financial stakes experienced by third parties will justify a substantial investment in case management in order to find a reasonable balance between care objectives and cost containment. Medicare could be a very important stimulus for the expansion of case management in home care if managed care continues to grow and if eligibility for home-care benefits is extended to include more disabled older people whose health care needs are less acute. In this instance, case managers will be needed who can balance health care and personal assistance objectives. Strong credentials in both health care and personal assistance will be needed for case managers in this arena.

Mahoney has identified ways in which independent case managers can plan a significant role in helping both clients and insurers to make the most effective use of equity that consumers build up when they purchase long-term care policies. They will be, it is believed, relieved of past conflicts of interest when case managers were employed by a provider who was interested in controlling spending. When clients build insurance equity, independent managers can help them plan their care to preserve that equity, which also is of value to insurers who will have to pay benefits as contracted for but can be assured that benefits are not wasted (Mahoney et al. 1996).

Private long-term case management will provide important opportunities and challenges for professionals. With the growth of the self-pay market and greater emphasis on self-direction among those with third-party financing, opportunities will be greatest for case managers who can persuade consumers that their services are worth the cost. The opportunities in this area are likely to be more narrowly focused and perhaps more often short-term than traditional case management.

The degree to which case management will develop as a professional specialty is uncertain. At present, social workers and community health nurses can move into supervisory positions in long-term care case management positions with modest in-service training and on-the-job training. The formation of a distinct professional specialization is more likely if the field grows substantially and becomes more complex. Closer ties between health care and personal assistance for the chronically ill in a managed-care environment, a wider range of community service options for long-term care clients living at home, more complex financing arrangements, greater responsibility on the part of case managers for client outcomes all point to greater professional specialization.

The manner in which private case managers develop their counseling role will influence the degree to which the field develops as a distinct profession. Case managers might offer comprehensive counseling on matters distinctive to long-term care. Such counseling would include advice to people in midlife about the risks associated with the eventual need for long-term care and assistance in advance planning for long-term care. Sound counseling in this arena requires thorough knowledge of private long-term care insurance options and basic understanding of estate planning and investment issues. In developing a comprehensive counseling practice, private case managers find it advantageous to work in collaboration with financial planners and lawyers who specialize in estate planning.

Similarly, private case mangers offering comprehensive counseling services would develop expertise in helping those who suddenly and unexpectedly become disabled and those with serious degenerating conditions to come to terms with their situation. This counseling would address psychological issues, interpersonal relations, family roles, and practical arrangements for living with disability. It would include knowledge of adaptive devices, knowledge of home modifications, and strategies for hiring and supervising personal assistants.

The degree to which various forms of private sector case management grow will depend on the ability of practitioners to sell their services to the self-pay consumer market and to insurance companies. The public that can afford to pay for services will have to be persuaded that expert advice is needed in negotiating long-term care options and that case managers specializing in home care are better sources of advice than physicians, lawyers, and more traditional nurses, and social workers.

In case management for home care, we are likely to have a mosaic of persons claiming professional expertise. They will include social workers and nurses for whom home care will be a specialty. They will be joined by others with different skills but without clinical training. Many will continue to have substantially less formal education. The field will be challenged to establish a coherent framework that finds a place for all of them and yet recognizes more complex skills when they are required.

In the long run, we may see affiliations emerge among various professions specializing in long-term care generally and home care more specifically. We anticipate increasing specialized expertise developing among those who administer programs that combine health care and personal assistance, architects specializing in home adaptations, hardware and software engineers concerned with adaptive technology, insurance professionals concerned with long-term care policies, lawyers involved with estate planning, and private case managers who work directly with clients and their families. Professionals in all of these fields who specialize in long-term care will recognize a need to keep abreast of developments involving other professions also involved with long-term care.

Medicine has seen such a proliferation of skill sets over its history, bound together by a focus on health care objectives and acceptance of basic universal practice standards. Home-care professionals will be challenged to develop a field with similar coherence. They have a great deal to accomplish in articulating widely shared objectives for the field that set it apart from health care. They will also have to demonstrate mastery over a set of skills that is persuasive to the fee-paying public, to other professionals and to third-parties sources of financing. The efforts of case managers in home care to professionalize represents a modest step in this direction. A great deal of intellectual and organizational energy will be required to achieve a distinctly defined home-care profession that is coherent in the manner in which it draws upon diverse specialties.

Conclusion

*T*HIS ANALYSIS concludes with a summary of our projections about the future of personal assistance and our proposals to strengthen its role in confronting long-term (lifelong) disability at all ages.

We began by examining the current status of personal assistance in long-term care. We propose that long-term care consists of three segments or phases: the first involves active but brief treatment, usually in a medical setting, and the second combines therapy with personal assistance, usually for several weeks or months as restoration of normal functioning is the major objective. In the third phase, the person's major need is for personal assistance because of serious, long-term functional limitations. In the third phase, individuals are usually living at home. In this phase, medical care is usually largely ameliorative. (See Figure 1 in Chapter 2.)

Life at home with functional disability usually requires personal help of some kind, care traditionally provided by family or friends. As family life has changed and technology in medical care has advanced, need for supplementary assistance from more formal arrangements has become more prevalent. Because current practices and policies have not developed to address this third phase fully, we find long-term care essentially an incomplete system in need of attention.

The 1990s transition in health policy and financing is a good time to pursue the completion of the role of long-term care. Our premise is that the objectives of health reform are not limited to cutting hospital and nursing home use in order to cut spending. They also include improving the opportunity for the chronically ill and functionally limited to approximate normal lives. A reordering of family, informal, and agency personal assistance joins medical care as central for completing the long term continuum.

Summary of the Analysis

1. The population dependent on some form of personal assistance is large, and expected to grow exponentially in the future because of demographic trends and life-sustaining scientific technology (Chapters 2 and 8).

2. Through Medicare and Medicaid, public policies have concentrated financing on the first and second phases, that is, mainly for the initial costs of medical and related rehabilitation interventions usually in a medical or nursing institution.

3. The emphasis on the medical end of the continuum has led to extensive use of institutions with high costs per patient (chaps. 5, 10).

4. In the postacute phase of health care, increasingly complex therapies are being provided in home settings.

5. Current public or collective arrangements for long-term care for those in the third phase with stable medical conditions and long-term disabilities are sharply limited.

6. Access to subsidized agency care services is limited to: (a) the poor and the nursing home eligible, including those who "spend down" to become eligible; (b) the elderly who are expected to be restored to health or function after a relatively brief period of posthospital therapy or who need continual but often intermittent medical procedures and attention at home, for which intermittent personal assistance is a minor adjunct; and (c) some of the very developmentally disabled.

7. The growing attention to prevention has concentrated on primary prevention by use of medical procedures, education for healthy life styles at younger ages, and the promises of gene therapy and early diagnoses of life threatening diseases. Secondary and tertiary prevention usually involve attention to the environment, including the home or institution as well as exposure to poisons and environmental hazards.

8. Efforts to discourage unnecessary institutional care and to encourage development of home and community-based services have been encouraged through Medicaid waivers.

9. Long-term life at home with self-care limitations requires personal assistance to complement residual physical capacities. Historically, this support has been left predominantly to families. In the judgment of many policy

makers and citizens, this reliance on families is appropriate. However, those who champion family responsibilities often have not confronted changes in family capacities and structure or the complexity of many disabilities with which they may have to cope.

10. Personal assistance services are in general provided by small, often specialized agencies with uncertain funding. They tend to be less effective than other interest groups in competing for public resources for services in the long-term care continuum.

11. Labor force of personal assistance and most home agencies is often viewed as unskilled. Because it is poorly paid and lacks a career ladder, it is difficult to recruit and retain workers competitively and efficiently.

12. Many states have been stimulated to develop modest programs that provide a variety of home- and community-based services at costs that are well below those of nursing home costs to those whose chronic illnesses and disabilities would qualify them for nursing home care.

    Lack of capital and limited experience in program development has limited such services in the ways they can serve those who pay for care themselves or whose care is financed through private insurance. Providers also are often limited (given the staff and resources available) in competitively offering services for the many varieties of specialized handicapping conditions, both physical and mental, which advances in medical science, in life extension, and in demography have created. The complexity of home care has increased more rapidly than the ability of small agencies to respond.

13. Resource constraints dictate a search for ways to extend the effectiveness of home care at modest cost. We should not anticipate any dramatic developments that will greatly increase the efficiency of home care. However, a number offer potential. Cash as an alternative to in-kind benefits in programs financed through third parties is currently attracting a good deal of attention (Chapter 5). For a well-informed consumer, cash can provide greater options in addressing personal assistance needs than a program that offers a limited menu of personal assistance options. If programs that offer cash benefits can reduce case management costs, some of the savings can also be used to expand benefits.

    Assistive devices represent an important resource for personal assistance (Chapter 6). Over time, extensive paid human assistance is inevitably expensive. Various mechanical and electrical devices cannot eliminate the need for human assistance, but they can sometimes reduce the need significantly. Personal response systems, for example, can provide access to emergency services at a modest cost. We suspect that the potential is great for effective deployment of many more assistive devices particularly among older personal assistance consumers who have not received occupational therapy services. We envision particular promise for low-cost devices that are not aggressively marketed. Assistive devices are a useful focus for consumer education.

Volunteers can enhance personal assistance services at modest cost (Chapter 7). Although the tradition of volunteering in the United States is strong, professionals are often skeptical about the value of volunteer contributions. The potential for greater involvement of volunteers in personal assistance services deserves careful consideration. Volunteers are unlikely candidates to perform core personal care tasks or major household tasks on a regular basis, but they can provide intermittent help and enrichment that personal assistance recipients often welcome. Volunteers, for example, can deliver meals, assist with shopping, deliver library books, help with transportation and escort, run errands, and simply visit. Volunteers, however, are not a free resource. Personal assistance providers who hope to use volunteers effectively must design volunteer projects carefully and systematically pursue recruitment, placement, training, supervision, and recognition of volunteers.

14. The greatest potential expansion for home care and for personal assistance will come from the large middle-income population that is economically independent. This population is increasingly aware of the need for personal assistants for relatives or, ultimately, for themselves and is already reaching out to alternatives to the nursing home solution.

Insurance in some form is attractive to this population, but few insurance products are available for personal assistance for long-term care. The families now caring for relatives at home are a major source of information about what future demand might be and their willingness or ability to pay to for it.

15. Changes in family structure have diminished the capacity of families to perform their former functions as primary providers of care at home by themselves. Families are smaller, and most adults work outside the home. Serial marriages increase the numbers of aged without close family. The numbers of lone individuals has not declined. As their relatives age, so do their children. Jobs take many of them far from their family base.

Until recently, advocates have expected that public services would eventually provide universal financing for long-term care, including home care. They expected that much of the extensive family role in long-term care could be shifted to a subsidized service. In the present political climate, introduction of a major new public program addressing personal assistance needs for those living in the community is most unlikely.

Economic trends have increased the financial capacity of middle-income families to plan for the future and also raised their living standards and expectations about family well-being. But the improved economic resources also improve the ability of middle-class families to finance their own long-term care.

16. The personal assistance field is poorly situated to meet the growing competition as new forms of institutional long-term care seem to be redefining what constitutes "a home": continuing care residential communities and assisted living facilities in many congregate forms have evolved to offer security, privacy, choice, and degrees of independent living in quasi congregate facilities. These packages give useful support services to fit individual needs.

17. Home care in any form has not yet developed ways to combine or package combinations of services at home, such as personal assistance, nurse aides, physical therapies, and some skilled nursing. This is now provided in poorly integrated ways by several kinds of service agencies through home health agencies for subacute care.

Personal assistance has a choice of remaining a minor subsidiary in the incomplete long-term care system or restructuring itself. This restructuring approach could also facilitate the growth of affordable insurance to cover personal assistance in true long-term home care. It would also position home care to reach out to the large population that may pay for personal assistance on an out-of-pocket basis.

18. Greater emphasis on self-financing of services and consumer control over long-term care financed by third parties (Chapter 5) will shift the discussion of balance between institutional and noninstitutional care. Institutional and noninstitutional providers will compete for clients or residents. Consumers will choose on the basis of their assessments of quality and cost.

Our analysis leaves us confronted with a puzzle. Consumers say they prefer home care to institutional care. Yet, aggregate spending for home care is modest. Consumer acceptance of formal home care seems to be greater when a third party pays for it. When they have the means, consumers seem more willing to pay substantial amounts for assisted living or nursing home care on an out-of-pocket basis. Several explanations are possible for the underspending on home care: (1) People prefer unpaid care by relatives; (2) consumers can get modest but adequate supplementary help at a modest price; (3) the formal agency help available is not seen as attractive enough to consumers to be worth paying for; (4) consumers have not learned that it may be sensible for them to make significant expenditures for personal assistance at home; (5) when need for help is great, consumers have more confidence in institutional services than in home care. Perhaps each accounts for some portion of the puzzle.

An important aspect of the puzzle involves insurance products. To what extent will policies be developed and be widely available that combine acceptable costs with strong personal assistance benefits? How will consumers respond? And, how will the personal assistance agencies respond to take advantage of such opportunities?

Home Care Allies

Home care has valuable allies in its attempts to deal with these weaknesses. Most obvious are the families and the handicapped themselves. Their effectiveness has been limited by absence of a common set of objectives, other than the expression of need and the reliance on more public funding for the economically dependent. In a time when public support for open generosity in tax funding is at a low ebb, they could be more effective if their goals were adjusted.

Younger disabled have already been articulate. They can be joined by many more from middle-class families that now provide most of the home care support themselves. Middle-class caregivers are beginning to recognize that there is no public backup for long-term care as we define it and are beginning to think about earlier planning for their own future needs, as well as for the more imminent needs of their still healthy elderly relatives. They can do this by earlier investing in better affordable home-care insurance policies, by assessing and reviewing possible reallocation of part of the disposable margin of their income for health needs, and by support of a completed, community-based, publicly financed long-term care system for the less affluent.

Proposals to Strengthen Home Care

The present weaknesses in personal assistance need to be approached at two levels with a clear conception about what a complete long-term care system entails: *completing* the system by strengthening support for those in the third phase of long-term care and *restructuring* personal assistance providers so that they are better able to serve both publicly and privately financed clients.

A major challenge for home care is to make itself attractive to economically independent consumers. Formal home care will have to compete with assisted living facilities and even with nursing homes. Can home care be organized more efficiently? Can it inspire greater confidence? Can its quality be improved so consumers with disabilities will purchase home care more often to complement informal (family) caregiving arrangements?

Our expectation is that any reconfiguration will be driven by such market forces more than by central planning efforts. Entrepreneurial personal assistance providers will experiment with various configurations. Such experimentation will go beyond new ways of deploying personal assistance staff; it may encompass assistive devices, differential use of informal help or of volunteers, architectural design for disabilities, and insurance brokers.

We suspect that two separate models will develop. Either model will be distinguished from the existing forms by some such phrase as "a comprehensive home care service" or "comprehensive services for care at home." One model will be built upon an expansion of the home health agency. Its centerpiece will be nursing, with physician and nurse practitioner backup. Aides will be deployed as personal assistance is needed. Unless federal polices are more radically changed than now seems likely, Medicare and Medicaid policies will dominate the evolution of this model. Health sector concentration is likely in this model because health and medical care needs are great and are backed by the extensive network of health providers and insurers, while personal assistance is subordinate: need for it is triggered by illness or injury. These providers need to organize themselves efficiently to offer their services at competitive prices and remember that personal assistance does not substitute for much in health care.

A second model, which might be called a broker model, emerges if personal assistance is dominant. We think that for a time it may consist of a loose configuration of personal assistance workers and case managers, either self-employed or employed in a variety of formal personal assistance agencies. These agencies may help clients and personal assistants in finding each other; they may help to administer wages and fringe benefits; they may help in household modification and in the use of assistive devices. Nursing will not be a significant part of this model, but nurse assistants will be. Case managers will be available to clients as consultants to assist in service planning. Case managers will encourage clients to consider a variety of strategies including personal assistance, home modification, and assistive devices. Case managers will also orchestrate volunteer services to provide welcome enhancements to complement family care and formal services. When asked to do so, case managers will also assist clients in finding other kinds of help that they need to remain independent, whether it is yard maintenance, home repair, or management of personal finances.

Financing for these services will be dominated by private payments, either through out-of-pocket payments or insurance. If the agency employs and deploys personal assistance workers, it will compete with independently employed workers and with assisted living facilities. It can serve a subsidized market of clients with limited means, but the major growth is not expected in services to low-income clients who require public financing.

Agencies of the first model can be major partners in health care; those of the second model will be more effective in serving a self-pay market. Not all agencies will be effective in pursuing both models. Some may be able to excel in both.

Consumer education is a major need for the personal assistance agency. Education includes sound information about how viable care at home can be arranged and managed by family and guidance about early purchase of insurance and what to look for in long-term care insurance policies.

More concretely, the central need is to restructure personal assistance services so that the field has units of sufficient scale to represent this end of the long-term care continuum effectively. Needed are agencies that offer comprehensive personal assistance services of high quality at modest prices, that can provide individual attention to diverse clients, that can develop skilled workers, and that can work with varied health, medical, and private insurance organizations as well as with families.

Such development needs professional leadership that can negotiate the ambiguous but interrelated boundaries between health and medical services and personal assistance services. Skilled professionals are also needed to negotiate the boundary between the care that families can provide and privately purchased supplemental help.

Personal assistance services must be restructured so that their scale of operation is expanded to the point that front line staff are able to perform varied tasks and their administrative staff are able to match those of more established institutions in terms of negotiating reimbursement policies with third parties and marketing to consumers. In one sense it means acquiring administrative staff who are credible in dealing with a highly bureaucratic world where large-scale organizations command expert negotiators. This is a challenge that confronts all nonprofit and for-profit human services.

Restructuring must also develop effective strategies for recruiting, training, and retaining a labor force capable of handling diverse personal care tasks and functions of care at home. Providers must be able to assure that their front-line staff can retain the confidence of patients and families whose needs are very diverse and individualized. Not all of these tasks require skilled medical or nursing personnel, but some of the tasks pose challenges that are beyond the capacities of many of the personnel who are currently in the labor force. These tasks also involve more skills than were required of the maid or caring relative in the historic model of family as care provider. This involves changing the boundaries of staff responsibilities.

Regional or urban manpower development is one possible approach to generating a sufficiently large and competent labor pool; such development is now beyond the capacities of small service agencies each trying to conduct its own training.

Restructuring must experiment with combinations of the two models to determine whether home care providers can be effective in fulfilling their responsibilities. Experimentation is also needed to determine if small agencies can survive by making highly efficient use of limited staff and collaborate effectively with other agencies offering complementary services.

Finally, restructuring should insure that agencies acquire the skills needed to market services effectively to self-financing middle-income populations.

How to Proceed

The field could wait for demand to entice numerous small local providers to develop new programs and see what results. We think this risky because the individual agencies lack the resources to respond to the changes in sight in any timely fashion. Other better-organized and better-capitalized programs, mainly medical and institutional, are in a good position to act first. If this happens, home care will remain a minor factor in long-term care. But there is no evidence that medically focused agencies will give the amount of attention to third-phase home care that the times require. Home care will be better served if providers whose central concern is personal assistance take the lead in developing more effective service models.

Personal assistance providers should collaborate in addressing certain common problems. For example, a regional labor force program is quite possible. Some of the other possibilities require capital and both personnel and fiscal resources that are now lacking. Still some collaboration is possible to employ specialized staff through umbrella organizations to handle specific joint ventures, such as marketing, negotiating public and private resource allocations, and developing entry into the large middle-income market represented by families with the functionally dependent at home. This requires more time and specialized skill than hard-pressed service managers may be able to give to be effective. Such skills can be acquired by an individual agency, but a consortium of agencies determined to build a system by collaboration is more likely to succeed. This approach demands that individual agencies concentrate on developing a system and a field, not a mosaic of agencies, by incremental changes in interagency cooperation.

Possibilities for expanded private investment to develop and market a strong personal assistance system should be explored. Substantial capital is already being invested in nursing homes and assisted living facilities. Similar investment might also be attracted to the development of stronger and profitable personal assistance services.

We recommend use of an old standby in times of transition—a national commission with major foundation funding. The commission would be charged to study the issues, develop a plan, and pursue the arduous task of persuading providers to implement the plan.

The 1950 National Commission on Chronic Illness was one such effort. It produced concepts that had an impact and are still useful. It did not address the organizational details, but there are successful examples of commissions that have set directions *and* formulated detailed implementation plans (see Morris and Binstock 1966). What is needed is leadership from some sources in the field, foundation backing (probably a consortium of foundations), and willingness of enough organizations in the field to join in. Such cooperation is common when it comes to accrediting agencies in a field. What we propose is more challenging, but not different in nature.

Through the means we have outlined, we urge the nation to complete the development of the long-delayed, truly long-term care system that will enable the most disabled to approximate normal lives in their own homes. It is possible for the nation to develop a system that will provide a more effective combination of personal, family, social, and medical services; that will strengthen the pursuit of personal assistance objectives when both medical care and personal assistance needs must be pursued; that will accept formal personal assistance as a complement to family caregiving; and that will acknowledge the limits of public responsibility.

Glossary

activities of daily living (ADLs) ADLs include: dressing, bathing, cooking, eating, toilet, etc.

assisted living, adult congregate housing, retirement housing, and independent living units Terms variously used to describe a multiple-unit apartment building in which the apartments all have bathrooms and kitchens, or kitchenettes, and where the management provides some supportive services, such as a dining room, optional housekeeping, transportation, and 24-hour watch service (Streib 1990).

continuing care (life care) retirement community (CCRC) An organization that offers a complete range of housing, residential services, and health care, from independent living to 24-hour skilled nursing care. CCRCs are notable in that they provide housing and health-related services for their residents under an agreement effective for the life of the resident or for a specific period.

formal care Social supports and assistance provided by someone who is *paid*, whether self-employed or employed by a private contractor, public agency, profit or nonprofit organization, or other service provider.

health care Those services and treatments recognized as contributing to physical or mental well-being, ranging from prevention to treatment and cure, including rehabilitation to restore function. Health care can be provided in most any setting: the home, place of employment, office of the provider, institution, etc.

health maintenance organization (HMO) An arrangement in which health services are provided to a voluntarily enrolled population within a specific geographic area. The providers are typically reimbursed on a capitated basis or through an "at risk" arrangement. There are a several different HMO models: staff, group, network, mixed, and independent practice association (IPA).

home health care The provision of medical care to someone living in their home or the community (e.g., nursing, speech therapy, intravenous drug therapy). Generally speaking, home health care is provided by someone who has been licensed or certified in a medical specialty.

hospice Care provided to terminally ill persons and their families that emphasizes emotional needs and coping with pain and death. It is a form of health care increasingly provided in a home setting.

informal care Social supports and assistance given by family members, friends, or volunteers

instrumental activities of daily living (IADLs) IADLs include: transportation, shopping, maintaining a checkbook, etc.

long-term care (LTC) A planned arrangement for the provision of personal assistance, medical care, and social supports required over a significant period of time by a functionally disabled person. Long-term care can be provided formally or informally at home, in the community, or in an institution

long-term care insurance This form of insurance is new but similar to other insurance in that it allows people to pay a known premium that offsets the risk of much larger out-of-pocket expenses. Several types of policy are available but most are "indemnity" policies, where they pay a fixed dollar amount for each day the insured receives care in either a nursing home or at home. Some life insurance policies offer long-term care benefits. Under these "accelerated" or "living benefits" provisions, a portion of the life insurance benefit is paid to the policy holder instead of the beneficiary at the policy-holder's death.

managed care A method of providing health care and services through financing mechanisms that coordinate care across time, place, and provider, emphasizing prevention, risk and reward sharing and appropriate utilization of services based on consumer and community needs for an outcome of maximum health and well-being at lower overall costs. Examples of managed care arrangements include: health maintenance organizations (HMOs), preferred provider organizations (PPOs), and points of service plans (POSs).

Medicaid (Title XIX of the Social Security Act, enacted 1965.) A federal- or state-funded program that pays the costs of health care provided for approximately 36 million low-income Americans. Medicaid serves multiple roles for the populations it covers. For example, in addition to paying for acute health care costs for eligible children and families, Medicaid pays for home health care, nursing home care, intermediate care facilities for the mentally retarded, and mental health care. Medicaid also pays Medicare premiums for low-income elderly persons, as well as special payments to hospitals that care for a disproportionately large share of uninsured individuals and Medicaid recipients.

medical care The term used to describe an array of interventions, treatments, or regimens authorized, coordinated, or provided by physicians, nurses, and other licensed health care professionals. Medical care may be labeled as inpatient or outpatient and it can be provided almost anywhere; however, its most difficult and intense practice is likely to be in a doctor's office, clinic, or hospital.

Medicare (Title XVIII of the Social Security Act, enacted 1965.) The nation's largest health insurance program. It covers nearly 34 million persons 65 and over and 5 million disabled persons. Medicare consists of two parts: Hospital Insurance (Part A) and Supplementary Medical Insurance (Part B). Medicare (Part A) covers home health care and hospice care, which can include personal assistance, in very limited circumstance and for brief periods. For all practical purposes, Medicare, like most health insurance, is not a financial resource for chronic illnesses or for long-term care.

nursing home or institutional care A congregate facility staffed and equipped to provide residents some type of 24-hour care. The care provided may be simply custodial (food, clothing, personal assistance, security) or it may include levels of care up to an and including skilled nursing care provided by a trained nurse, physical therapist, or other professional health care provider

Older Americans Act A federal categorical grant program through which public funds are distributed to states and area agencies on aging (AAA). Older Americans Act funds support senior centers, congregate and delivered meals programs, information and referral networks, nursing home ombudsman services, day care, respite programs, and other supportive services designed to help older persons remain in independent living status as long as possible.

personal assistance or personal care The help provided a functionally disabled person who cannot manage independently all the activities of daily living (ADL). Personal care can be provided in most any setting, either formally or informally.

points-of-service plans (POSs) POSs offer a full range of health services through a combination of HMO and PPO features.

preferred provider organization (PPO) An arrangement through which the sponsoring group negotiates price discounts with providers in exchange for patients. The sponsor may be an insurer, employer, or third-party administrator.

rehabilitation The term given to a process of restoring disabled persons to maximum physical, mental, and vocational independence and productivity.

residential care facilities A term used to describe an array of housing options including: assisted living, adult group homes, board and care homes, domiciliary care, family care, and rest homes. The general characteristics of residential care facilities are: the rooms are usually rented, housekeeping services are provided, meals served in a central dining area, personal assistance available, and 24-hour security.

reverse home mortgage An instrument that allows older people to realize the financial equity in their home without selling it. With a reverse mortgage, the older homeowner is allowed to borrow from the equity value in their home, receiving a predetermined set of monthly cash payments over some defined period.

social/health maintenance organization (S/HMO) A federally supported demonstration of a single entry, prepaid, long-term care service delivery model in which one organization takes the lead in financing and coordinating a range of medical and nonmedical home care services not ordinarily covered by Medicare or other supplemental health insurance plans.

Social Services Block Grant (Title XX of the Social Security Act, 1975.) A program by which the national government distributes to the states more than $2.5 billion to be used to help needy persons achieve economic self-support or personal self-sufficiency. Title XX funds are used by many states to provide personal care services to functionally disabled persons and others at risk of institutionalization.

social supports, supportive services, social services The provision of housing, transportation, congregate or delivered meals, day care, homemaker, chore services, and other programs or activities designed to enhance the quality of life.

References

AARP (American Association of Retired Persons). 1988. "National Survey of Caregivers." Washington, D.C.: American Association of Retired Persons.

Aetna Life Insurance Company. "Long-term Care: Introduction to Aetna's Employer Sponsored Group Long-term Care Insurance Plan." Hartford, Conn.

Agree, E. M. 1994. "The Role of Technology in Long-Term Care: Preliminary Results from the Survey of Asset and Health Dynamics of the Oldest-Old (AHEAD)." Presented at the AHEAD early results workshop, Ann Arbor.

Alley, J. M. 1988. "Family Caregiving: Family Strains, Coping Response, Patterns, and Caregiver Burden." Ph.D. diss., Virginia Polytechnic University.

American Association of Homes and Services for the Aging. 1990. *Understanding Senior Housing for the 1990s.* Washington, D.C.: American Association of Retired Persons.
———. 1997. Washington, D.C.

American Health Care Association. 1995. *Facts and Trends: The Nursing Facility Fact Book.* Washington, D.C.: American Health Care Association.

Andersen, R. M. 1995. "Revisiting the Behavioral Model and Access to Medical Care: Does It Matter?" *Journal of Health and Social Behavior* 36:1–10.

Assisted Living Facilities Association of America. 1993. *Assisted Living Facilities in America 1993.* Fairfax, Va.

Bader, J. E. 1994. *Assistive ("Prosthetic") Devices.* Long Beach: Center for Successful Aging, California State University.

Banazak-Holl, J., and M. A. Hines. 1996. "Factors Associated with Nursing Home Staff Turnover." *Gerontologist* 36, no. 4: 512–17.

Bardwell, F. 1930. "Public Outdoor Relief and Care of the Aged in Massachusetts." In M. Rubinow, ed., *Care of the Aged.* Chicago: University of Chicago Press.

Batavia, A. I., and G. DeJong. 1990. "Developing a Comprehensive Health Services Research Capacity in Physical Disability and Rehabilitation." *Journal of Disability Policy Studies* 1:37–61.

Bayer, Ron, and E. Feldman. 1985. "Hospice under Medicare Wing." *Report 12 (6).* Hastings, N.Y.: Hastings Center.

Beland, F. 1984. "The Decision of Elderly Persons to Leave Their Homes." *Gerontologist* 24:179–85.

Benjamin, A. E. 1993. "An Historical Perspective on Home Care Policy." *Milbank Quarterly* 71, no. 1: 129–66.

Berkowitz, Edward. 1997. "Research and Politics in Policy Making for Social Security." *Journal of Gerontology: Social Sciences* 52B, no. 3: S115–24.

Biaggi, M. 1980. *Testimony before the Select Committee on Aging.* Washington, D.C.: House of Representatives, 96th Congress.

Binstock, R. H., L. E. Cluff, and O. von Mering, eds. 1996. *The Future of Long-term Care: Social and Policy Issues.* Baltimore: Johns Hopkins University Press.

Blanchette, K. 1997. *New Directions for Long Term Care Systems.* Vol. 3: *Supporting.* Washington, D.C.: Public Policy Institute of the American Association of Retired Persons.

Boas, E. 1930. "Care of the Aged Sick." In I. M. Rubinow, ed., *Care of the Aged.* Chicago: University of Chicago Press.

Boaz, R., and J. Hu. 1997. "Determining the Amount of Help Used by Disabled Elderly Persons at Home: The Role of Coping Resources." *Journal of Gerontology: Social Sciences* 52B, no. 6: S317–24.

Boaz, R., and C. Muller. 1994. "Predicting the Risk of 'Permanent' Nursing Home Residence: The Role of Community Help as Indicated by Family Helpers and Prior Living Arrangements." *Health Services Research* 29:391–414.

Bowe, F. 1989. "Why Seniors Don't Use Technology." *Technology Review* August–September, 34.

Boyd, Bruce. 1990. "Long-term Care: It's Your Choice." *Generations* 1 (Spring): 23–27.

Brakman, S. V. 1994. "Adult Daughter Caregivers." *Hastings Center Report* 24:26–28.

Brecher, C., and J. Knickman. 1985. "A Reconsideration of Long-term Care Policy." *Journal of Health, Politics, Policy and Law* 10, no. 2: 245–73.

Brecher, C., J. Knickman, and R. Vogel. 1986. "Local Simulations of Alternative Policies for Financing Services to the Elderly." *Medical Care* 24, no. 4: 363–76.

Breen, Thomas. 1992. "Community Alarm Systems." *Home Health Care Services Quarterly* 13, nos. 3–4: 191–99.

Brody, E. M. 1981. "Women in the Middle and Family Help to Older People." *Gerontologist* 27:259–65.

Burbridge, L. C. 1993. "The Labor Market for Home Care Workers: Demand, Supply and Institutional Barriers." *Gerontologist* 33:41–46.

Callahan, James. 1989. "Case Management for the Elderly: A Panacea?" *Journal of Aging and Social Policy* 1:181–85.

———. 1996. "Care in the Home and Other Community Settings: Present and Future." In R. H. Binstock, L. E. Cluff, and O. von Mering, eds., *The Future of Long-term Care: Social and Policy Issues.* Baltimore: Johns Hopkins University Press.

Callander, Marie, and J. Lavor. 1975. "Home Care Development, Problems, and Potentials." Washington, D.C.: U.S. Department of Health, Education, and Welfare.

Cameron, K. A., and J. P. Firman. 1995. "International and Domestic Programs Using Cash and Counseling: Strategies to Pay for Long-Term Care." *Draft Report* (March). Washington, D.C.: National Council on the Aging.

Cantor, M. 1992. "Families and Caregiving in an Aging Society." *Generations* 16 (Summer): 67–70.

Caro, Frank. 1973. "Personal Care Organization." Working Papers. Levinson Policy Institute. Waltham: Brandeis University.

Caro, F. G. 1986. "Relieving Informal Caregiver Burden through Organized Services." In

K. A. Pillemer and R. Wolf, eds., *Elder Abuse: Conflict in the Family.* Dover, Mass.: Auburn House.

Caro, F. G., and A. E. Blank. 1988. *Quality Impact of Home Care for the Elderly* New York: Haworth Press.

Caro, Francis, and Robert Morris. 1995. "Retraining Older Workers: An Emerging Need." *American Community College Journal* 63, no. 3: 22–26.

Caro, F., and S. Bass. 1992. "Patterns of Productive Aging." Gerontology Institute. Boston: University of Massachusetts–Boston.

Caro, F., and S. Bass. 1995. "Dimensions of Productive Engagement." In S. Bass, ed., *Older and Active,* 204–16. New Haven: Yale University Press.

Chambers, Clark. 1963. *Seed Time of Reform.* Minneapolis: University of Minnesota Press.

Chen, Y.-P. 1993. "A Three-legged Stool: A New Way to Fund Long-term Care?" *Care in the Long Term.* Washington, D.C.: National Academy Press, Institute of Medicine.

Chichin, E. 1989. "Community Care for the Frail Elderly: The Case of Non-professional Home Care Workers." In L. Grau and I. Susser, eds., *Women in the Later Years: Health, Social, and Cultural Perspectives.* New York: Haworth Press.

Clark, J. 1996. *California Long-Term Care Insurance Policy Comparison Chart.* Huntington Beach, Calif.: Retired Employees Association of Orange County.

Cohen, M. A., N. Kumar, and T. McGuire. 1991. "Long Term Care Financing Proposals." *HIAA Research Bulletin.* Washington, D.C.: Health Insuarance Association of America.

Coleman, Barbara. 1996. *New Directions for State and Long-term Care Systems.* Vol. 1. Washington, D.C.: Public Policy Institute of the American Association of Retired Persons.

Coleman, K., and J. Kiefer. 1986. "The Older Volunteer Resource." In *America's Aging: Productive Roles in an Aging Society.* Washington, D.C.: National Academy Press, Institute of Medicine.

Coll, Blanche D. 1995. *Safety Net: Welfare and Social Security 1929–1979.* New Brunswick: Rutgers University Press.

Collins, C., and M. Stommel. 1991. "Out-of-pocket Expenditures by Family Caregivers of Dementia Patients Residing in the Community." *Home Health Care Services Quarterly* 12, no. 4: 29–43.

Commonwealth Fund. 1993. "The Untapped Resource: Final Report of the American over 55 at Work Program." *Report* 66. New York: Commonwealth Fund.

Congressional Budget Office (CBO). 1977. "Long-Term Care Actuarial Estimates." Washington, D.C.

Congressional Quarterly Weekly. 1997. 55, no. 31 (Aug. 2): 1144.

Crown, W., J. Capitman, and W. Leutz. 1992. "Economic Rationality, the Affordability of Private Long-term Care Insurance, and the Role of Public Policy." *Gerontologist* 32: 478–85.

Crown, W., M. MacAdam, and E. Sadowsky. 1991 "Health Aides Characteristics and Working Conditions of Aides Working in Hospitals, Nursing Homes and Home Care." Report to Health Care Financing Administration for Home Care Quality Project. Bigel Institute. Waltham: Brandeis University.

Crown, W., J. Capitman, and W. Leutz. 1992. "Economic Rationality, the Affordability of Private Long-term Care Insurance, and the Role of Public Policy." *Gerontologist* 32: 478–85.

Derthick, M. 1975. *Uncontrollable Spending for Social Services.* Washington, D.C.: Brookings Institution.

———. 1990. *Aging under Stress: The Social Security System Administration in America.* Washington, D.C.: Brookings Institution.

Dibner, Andrew S. 1992. "Personal Response Systems: Present and Future." *Home Health Care Services Quarterly* 13, nos. 3–4: 239–43.

Doty, P. 1986. "Family Care of the Elderly: The Role of Public Policy." *Milbank Quarterly* 64:34–75.

Doty, P., J. Kasper, and S. Litvak. 1991. "Consumer Directed Models of Personal Care: Lessons from Medicaid." *Milbank Quarterly* 74, no. 3.

Doty, P., and B. Miller. 1993. "Caregiving and Productive Aging." In S. Bass, F. Caro, and Y.-P. Chen, eds., *Achieving a Productive Aging Society,* 143–66. Westport, Conn.: Auburn House.

Eggert, Gerald, et al. 1977. "Caring for the Patient with Long Term Disability." *Geriatrics* 32, no. 10: 3–20.

Enders, A. 1986. "Issues and Options in Technology for Disability and Aging." In C. W. Mahoney, C. L. Estes, and J. E. Heumann, eds., *Toward a Unified Agenda: Proceedings of a National Conference on Disability and Aging.* San Francisco: Institute for Health and Aging, University of California, San Francisco.

Epstein, A. 1930. "Facing Old Age." In I. M. Rubinow, ed., *Care of the Aged.* Chicago: University of Chicago Press.

Estes, C., and E. A. Binney. 1988. "Toward a Transformation of Health and Aging Policy." University of California, San Francisco. Institute on Health and Aging.

Families USA Foundation. 1994. *Doing Without: The Sacrifices Families Make to Provide Home Care.* Number 94-107. Washington, D.C.: Families USA.

Feder, Judith. 1991. "Paying for Home Care: The Limits of Current Programs." In D. Rowland and B. Lyons, eds., *Financing Home Care: Improving Protection for Disabled Elderly People,* 27–47. Baltimore: Johns Hopkins University Press.

Feldman, P. H. 1988. *Who Cares for the Workers in the Home Care Industry?* San Francisco: Greenwood.

Feldman, P. H., R. Sapienza, and R. Kane. 1993. "Work Life Improvements for Health Care Workers." *Geriatrics* 33:47–54.

Firman, J. 1983. "Reforming Community Care for the Elderly and Disabled." *Health Affairs* 2 (Spring): 66–82.

Follman, J. F., Jr. 1963. *Medical and Health Insurance: A Study in Social Progress.* Homewood, Ill.: Richard D. Irwin.

Frazer, I. l985. "Medicare Reimbursement for Hospice Care: Ethical and Policy Implications of Cost Containment Strategies." *Journal of Health Politics* 10, no. 3: 565–78.

Glickman, L., K. Stocker, and F. Caro. 1997. "Self Direction in Home Care for Older People: A Consumer's Perspective." *Home Health Care Services Quarterly* 16, nos. 1–2: 41–54.

Government Accounting Office. 1992. "Long-Term Care Insurance: Better Controls Needed in Sales to People with Limited Financial Resources." GAO/HRD-92-66. Washington, D.C.: U.S. Government Printing Office.

Grana, J. 1983. "Disability Allowances for Long-term Care in Western Europe and the United States." *International Social Security* 36, no. 2: 207–21.

Gratton, Brian. 1997. "The Politics of Dependency Estimates: Social Security Board Estimates, 1935–1939." *Journal of Gerontology: Social Science* 52B: S117–24.

Greene, V. L., M. E. Lovely, and J. J. Ondrich. 1993. "Do Community-based, Long-term Care Services Reduce Nursing Home Use?" *Journal of Human Resources* 28:297–317.

Gruenberg, F. 1994. "The Failures of Success." *National Health Expenditures.* Baltimore: Health Care Financing Administration.

Gruenberg, L., and L. Pillemer. 1981. "Disability Allowances for Long Term Care." In J. Callahan and S. Wallack, eds., *Reforming the Long Term Care System.* University Health Policy Center, Brandeis. Lexington, Mass.: Lexington Books.

Gruman, C. 1997. *An Analyis of Case Management Programs and Practices: Correlates of Organizational Strength.* Ph.D. diss., University of Massachusetts–Boston.

Hansan, John E. 1980. *A Study of State Government Decision Making in the Allocation of Title XX Funds.* Ph.D. diss., Florence Heller School, Brandeis University, Waltham.

Hansan, John E., and Robert Morris. 1997 "A Decade Long Drift to Public Conservatism: Redefining the Federal Roles in Social Welfare." In John E. Hansan and Robert Morris, eds., *The National Government and Social Welfare: What Should Be the Federal Role?* Westport, Conn.: Greenwood Publishing Group.

Harrow, B., S. Tennstedt, and J. McKinlay, 1995. "How Costly Is It to Care for Disabled Elders in a Community Setting?" *Gerontologist* 35, no. 6: 3–13.

Haslanger, K. 1995. "Is Case Management of Any Value? What Is the Evidence?" *Journal of Long-term Home Health Care* 14 no. 2: 37–43.

Hatch, R. C., and M. C. Franken. 1984. "Concerns of Children with Parents in Nursing Homes." *Journal of Gerontological Social Work* 7:19–30.

Health Care Financing Administration. 1995. *Role of Medicare and Medicaid in Long Term Care: Opportunities, Challenges and New Directions.* Baltimore: Health Care Financing Administration.

———. 1996. *Your Medicare Handbook.* Washington, D.C.: U.S. Government Printing Office.

Herzog, A. R., and M. Morgan. 1993. "Formal Volunteer Work among Older Americans." In Scott Bass, Francis Caro, and Y. P. Chen, eds., *Achieving a Productive Aging Society.* Westport, Conn.: Auburn House.

Hijjazi, K. (1997). "Factors Contributing to Variations in Medicare Home Health Agency Services Utilization Among Aged Medicare Beneficiaries: Testing Alternate Models." Ph.D. diss., University of Massachusetts–Boston.

Hooyman, N. R., and A. H. Kiyak. 1993. *Social Gerontology: A Multidisciplinary Perspective.* 3d ed. Boston: Allyn & Bacon.

Hughes, S. L. 1985. "Apples and Oranges? A Review of Evaluations of Community-based Long-term Care." *Health Services Research* 20:461–88.

Hunt, Michael E. 1987. "Naturally Occurring Retirement Communities: A Model of Supportive Housing and Services for the Elderly." *Final Report.* Institute on Aging. Madison: University of Wisconsin.

Jarret, M. C. 1933. "Chronic Illness in New York City." *The Problems of Chronic Illness New York City,* vol. 1. New York: Columbia University Press.

Jarret, Mary. 1933. "Chronic Illness in New York City: The Care of the Sick by Different Types of Voluntary Agencies." *The Problems of Chronic Illness New York City,* vol. 2. New York: Columbia University Press.

Johansson, L., and M. Thorslund. 1993. "Care of the Elderly in Sweden—Formal and Informal Support." In F. Lesemann and C. Martin, eds., *Home-Based Care, the Elderly, the Family, and the Welfare State: An International Comparison.* Ottawa: University of Ottawa.

Kane, Rosalie, and Karen D. Wilson. 1993. *Assisted Living in the U.S.: A New Paradigm for Older Persons.* Washington, D.C.: American Association of Retired Persons.

Kassner, Enid, and J. Martin. 1996. "Decisions, Decisions: Service Based Allocations in Home and Community Based Long-Term Care Programs." October. Washington, D.C.: American Association of Retired Persons.

Kaye, L., and J. K. Davitt. 1995. "Provider and Consumer Profiles of Traditional and Hi-Tech Home Health Care." *Health and Social Work* 20, no. 4: 262–72.

Kemper, P., and C. M. Murtaugh. 1991. "Lifetime Use of Nursing Home Care." *New England Journal of Medicine* 324, no. 9: 595–600.

Kemper, P. 1992. "The Use of Formal and Informal Home Care by the Disabled." *Health Services Research* 27:421–51.

Knee, Ruth, and W. Lamson. 1971. "Mental Health Services." In *Encyclopedia of Social Work,* ed. Robert Morris. New York: National Association of Social Workers.

LaPlante, M. P. 1991. *Disability in Basic Life Activities across the Lifespan.* (Disability Statistics Report I). Washington, D.C.: National Institute of Disability and Rehabilitation Research.

Lavor, Judy. 1979. "Long Term Care: A Challenge to Service Systems." In V. LaPorte and J. Rubin, eds., *Reform and Regulation of Long Term Care.* New York: Praeger.

Lawton, M. P., E. M. Brody, and A. R. Saperstein. 1989. "Controlled Study of Respite Service for Caregivers of Alzheimer's Patients." *Gerontologist* 29:8–16.

Lesemann, F., and C. Martin. 1993. "Concluding Comments." In F. Lesemann and C. Martin, eds., *Home-Based Care, the Elderly, the Family, and the Welfare State: An International Comparison.* Ottawa: University of Ottawa.

Leutz, Walter. 1995. Exchange of letters re: S/HMO. *Gerontologist* 35, no. 3: 292–95.

Leutz, W., M. Greenlick, and J. Capitman. 1994. "Capitation: Integrating Acute and Long Term Care." *Health Affairs* 13, no. 4: 58–74.

Linsk, N., S. Kreigher, and L. Simon-Rusinowitz. 1992. *Wages for Caring.* New York: Praeger Press.

Lipson, D., and E. Donohoe. 1988. "State Financing of Long-Term Care Services for the Elderly." Intergovernmental Health Policy Project. Washington, D.C.: George Washington University.

Litvak, S., J. Heumann, and H. Zukas. 1987. "Attending to America: Personal Assistance for Independent Living: National Survey of Attendant Programs in the U.S." Washington, D.C.: World Institute on Disability.

Litwak, E. 1985. *Helping the Elderly: The Complementary Roles of Informal Networks and Formal Systems.* New York: Guilford Press.

Liu, K., K. G. Manton, and B. M. Liu. 1985. "Home Care Expenses for the Disabled Elderly." *Health Care Financing Review* 7, no. 2: 51–58.

Lubov, Roy. 1962. *The Progressives and the Slums.* Pittsburg: University of Pittsburg Press.

Lynn, J. 1996. "Caring at the End of Our Lives." *New England Journal of Medicine* 335, no. 3: 201–3.

MacAdam, Margaret. 1993. "Home Care Reimbursement and Effects on Personnel." *Gerontologist* 33:55–63.

Mahoney, K., et al. 1996. "Case Management for Private Payers." *Review of Gerontology and Geriatrics* 16:140–61.

Maslow, K., and J. O'Keeffe. 1998. *What Criteria Should Be Used to Determine Eligibility for Long Term Care Services: A Policy Framework.* Washington, D.C.: American Association of Retired Persons, forthcoming.

Master, Robert, et al. 1996. "The Community Medical Alliance: An Integrated System of Care in Boston for People with Severe Disabilities and AIDS." *Managed Care Quarterly* 4, no. 2: 26–37.

Mauser, E., and N. Miller. 1994. "A Profile of Home Health Care Users in 1992." *Health Care Financing Review* 16, no. 1: 17–33.

McArthur, John H., and Francis D. Moore. 1997. "The Two Cultures and the Health Care Revolution." *Journal of the American Medical Association* 277 (March): 985–89.

Meiners, M. R. 1984. "The State of the Art in Long-Term Care Insurance." Rockville: National Center for Health Services Research.

Meltzer, J. 1988. *Completing the Long-term Care Continuum: An Income Support Strategy.* Washington, D.C.: Center for Social Policy.

Moen, P., J. Robison, and V. Fields. 1994. "Women's Work and Caregiving Roles: A Life Course Approach." *Journal of Health and Social Behavior* 49:S176–S186.

Montgomery, Christina. 1992. "Personal Response Systems in the United States." *Home Health Care Services Quarterly* 13, nos. 3–4: 201–22.

Morgan, J. 1983. "Value of Volunteer Time." In G. Duncan and J. Morgan, eds., *Five Thousand American Families: Patterns of Economic Progress,* vol. 10. Ann Arbor: Institute for Social Research, University of Michigan.

Morris, Robert. 1961. "The Future Institution for the Aged." In *Reports and Guidelines for the White House Conference on Aging,* 99–109. Washington, D.C.: U.S. Department of Health, Education and Welfare.

———. 1971. *Alternatives to Nursing Home Care: A Proposal to the Senate Special Committee on Aging.* Washington, D.C.: U.S. Government Printing Office.

———. 1973. "What to Do When the Doctor Leaves." *Harper's Magazine,* January.

———. 1995. "Using Retirees to Address Social Ills." *Aging International* 22, no. 3: 16–23.

Morris, R., and R. H. Binstock. 1966. *Feasible Planning for Social Change.* New York and London: Columbia University Press.

Morris, Robert, and Francis Caro. 1995. "The Young-Old, Productive Aging, and Public Policy. *Generations* 19, no. 1: 32–38.

———. 1996. "Productive Retirement: Stimulating Greater Volunteer Efforts to Meet National Needs." *Journal of Volunteer Administration* 14, no. 2: 5–13.

Motenko, A. 1989. "Frustrations, Gratifications, and Well-being of Dementia Caregivers." *Gerontologist* 29, no. 2: 166–72.

National Alliance for Caregiving and American Association of Retired Persons. 1997. *Family Caregiving in the U.S.: Findings from a National Survey.* Bethesda: National Alliance for Caregiving.

National Commission on Chronic Illness. 1956. *Care for the Long-Term Patient.* Cambridge: Harvard University Press.

National Conference of State Legislatures. 1997. *Task Force Report.* Denver: National Conference of State Legislatures.

National Council on Disability. 1993. *Study on the Financing of Assistive Technology Devices and Services for Individuals with Disabilities.* Washington, D.C.: National Council on Disability.

Neuschler, E. 1987. *Medicaid Eligibles Need Long Term Care.* Washington, D.C.: National Governors Conference.

New York Times. April 18, 1996. "City Pledges to Enhance Home Care for Elderly."

Newman, Sandra, and K. Envall. 1995. *Effects of Supports on Sustaining Older Persons in the Community.* Washington, D.C.: American Association of Retired Persons.

Pepper Commission. 1990. *A Call for Action.* Washington, D.C.: U.S. Government Printing Office.

Persons in the Community. AARP. Washington, September 1995 Older Americans Report 1986. Washington, D.C.: U.S. Department of Health and Human Services, Administration on Aging.

Phillips, Harry. 1971. "Disability and Handicap." In *Encyclopedia of Social Work,* ed. Robert Morris. New York: National Association of Social Workers.

Pillemer, K. A., and R. Wolf, eds. 1986. *Elder Abuse: Conflict in the Family.* Dover, Mass.: Auburn House.

Pynoos, J., and S. Golant. 1995. "Housing and Living Arrangements for the Elderly." In R. H. Binstock and L. K. George, eds., *Handbook of Aging and Social Sciences,* 303–24. 4th ed. San Diego: Academic Press.

Risse, G. B., R. L. Numbers, and J. W. Leavitt, eds. 1977. *Medicine without Doctors: Home Health Care in American History.* New York: Science History Publications.

Rivlin, A. M, and J. M. Wiener. 1988. *Caring for the Disabled Elderly: Who Will Pay?* Washington, D.C.: Brookings Institution.

Rosenberg, Connie. 1995. "Controversies in Case Management." *Journal of Long-Term Home Health Care* 14, no. 3: 37–42.

Rossi, A. S. and P. H. Rossi. 1990. *Of Human Bonding: Parent-child Relations across the Life Course.* New York: A. de Gruyter.

Rothman, David. 1956. *Discovery of Asylum: Care for the Long-Term Patient.* Cambridge: Harvard University Press.

Rowland, D., and B. Lyons. 1990. *Living Alone with Disability: Home Care Use and Burdens.* Department of Health Policy and Management, School of Hygiene and Public Health. Baltimore: Johns Hopkins University Press.

Ruchlin, Hirsch S., and John Morris. 1981. "Cost Benefit Analysis of an Emergency Alarm and Response System: A Case Study of a Long-term Care Program." *Health Services Research* 16, no. 1: 65–80.

Sabatino, C. 1990. *Lesson for Enhancing Consumer-Directed Approaches in Home Care.* January. New York: Commonwealth Fund.

Sager, Alan. 1976. Testimony before the Senate Special Committee on Aging on S.B. 575. Levinson Policy Institute. Waltham: Brandeis University.

Salmen, John P. 1994. *The Do-Able Renewable Home: Making Your Home Fit Your Needs.* Washington, D.C.: American Association of Retired Persons.

Salmons, T. 1996. "Predicting a Future Need for Long-term Care: The Influence of Parents' Experiences." M.A. thesis, University of Massachusetts–Boston.

Scanlon, W., 1992. "Possible Reforms for Financing Long-term Care." *Journal of Economic Perspectives* 6, no. 3: 43–58.

Scholen, K., and Y.-P. Chen, eds. 1980. *Unlocking Home Equity for the Elderly.* Cambridge: Ballinger.

Seeleman, K. D. 1993. "Assistive Technology Policy: A Road to Independence for Individuals with Disabilities." *Journal of Social Issues* 49, no. 2: 115–36.

Shapiro, J. P. 1994. "Death on Trial: The Case of Dr. Kevorkian Obscures Critical Issues." *U.S. News and World Report* 116, no. 16: 31–37.

Sherwood, Sylvia, and John Morris. 1980. *A Study of an Emergency Alarm and Response System for the Aged: A Final Report.* Rockville: National Center for Health Services Research.

Sherwood, Sylvia, et al. 1997. *Continuing Care Retirement Communities.* Baltimore: Johns Hopkins University Press.

Short, P. F., and J. Leon. 1990. "Use of Home and Community Services by Persons Age 65 and Older with Functional Difficulties." *National Medical Expenditures Survey—Research Findings.* U.S. Department of Health and Human Services. Washington, D.C.: Government Printing Office.

Silvestri, George. 1993. "The American Work Force, 1992–2005." *Monthly Labor Review* 116, no. 11: 58–86.

Social Security Administration. 1996. *Income of the Aged: Chartbook, 1994.* Baltimore: Office of Research and Statistics.

Spann, Jerry. 1987. *The Community Options Program.* Madison: LaFollette Institute of Public Affairs, University of Wisconsin.

Statistical Abstract of the United States. 1994. Washington, D.C.: U.S. Department of Commerce, Bureau of Census. Tables 169, 639.

Stern, A. L. 1995. *A Multidimenional Assessment of Caregiving Outcomes.* Ph.D. diss., University of Massachusetts–Boston.

Stoller, E. P., and S. J. Cutler. 1993. "Predictors of Use of Paid Help among Older People Living in the Community." *Gerontologist* 33:31–40.

Stone, R. I., and P. Kemper. 1989. "Spouses and Children of Disabled Elderly: How Large a Constituency for Long-term Reform?" *Milbank Quarterly* 67:485–506.

Stum, M. S., J. W. Bauer, and P. J. Delaney. 1996. "Out-of-pocket Home Care Expenditures for Disabled Elderly." *Journal of Consumer Affairs* 30, no. 1: 24–47.

Sung, K. 1994. "Measures and Dimensions of Filial Piety in Korea." *Gerontologist* 35, no. 2: 240–47.

Suzman, R., and K. Manton. 1992. "Forecasting Health and Functioning in Aging Societies." In M. G. Orly, P. Abeles, and P. D. Lipman, eds., *Aging, Health, and Behavior.* Newbury Park, Calif.: Sage Publications.

Tennstedt, S. L., S. Crawford, and J. B. McKinlay. 1993a. "Determining the Pattern of Community Care: Is Coresidence More Important than Caregiver Relationship?" *Journal of Gerontology* 48: S74–83.

———. 1993b. "Is Family Care on the Decline? A Longitudinal Investigation of the Substitution of Formal Long-term Care Services for Informal Care." *Milbank Quarterly* 71:601–22.

Thurow, L. 1974. "Cash versus In-Kind Transfers." *American Economic Review* 64, no. 2: 190–95.

Treas, J. 1995. "Older Americans in the 1990s and Beyond." *Population Bulletin* 50, no. 2: 1–43.

U.S. Bureau of the Census. 1995. Statistical Brief. S.B./95-8. *Sixty Five Plus in the U.S.* Washington, D.C.: U.S. Department of Commerce.

U.S. Bureau of the Census. 1996. "Population in the U.S. over Age 65." In *Current Populations Reports: Special Studies,* 23–190. Washington, D.C.: U.S. Department of Commerce.

U.S. Department of Health and Human Services. 1990. *Survey of Income and Program Participation.* Washington, D.C.: U.S. Government Printing Office.

U.S. Department of Labor, Bureau of Labor Statistics. 1990. *Outlook 2000.* Bulletin 2352. Washington, D.C.: U.S. Government Printing Office.

U.S. Senate Special Committee on Aging. 1992. *Aging America: Trends and Projections.* Washington, D.C.: U.S. Government Printing Office.

U.S. Senate Special Committee on Aging. 1996. *Long Term Challenge: Developments in Aging,* vol. 3. Washington, D.C.: Government Printing Office.

UNUM Life Insurance Company of America, Individual Long-term Care Policy Information. Portland, Maine.

Vladeck, B. C. 1980. *Unloving Care: The Nursing Home Tragedy.* New York: Basic Books.

———. 1995. "End of Life Care." *Journal of the American Medical Association* 274, no. 6: 449.

Weissert, W. 1985. "Home and Community Based Care: The Cost Effectiveness Trap." *Generations* 10:47–50.

———. 1988a. "National Channeling Demonstration: What We Knew, What We Know Now, and Need to Know." *Health Services Research* 23, no. 1: 175–87. Washington, D.C.: U.S. Government Printing Office.

———. 1988b. "Size and Characteristics of the Noninstitutional Long-term Care Population." In *Project to Analyze Existing Long-term Care Data,* vol. 2, *The Long Term Care Population.* Washington, D.C.: The Urban Institute.

———. 1991. "A New Policy Agenda for Home Care." *Health Affairs* 10:67–77.

Weissert, W. G., C. M. Cready, and J. E. Pawelak. 1988. "The Past and Future of Home and Community Based Long-term Care." *Milbank Quarterly* 66:309–88.

White, G. W., et al. 1996. "Preventing and Managing Secondary Conditions: A Proposal for Centers for Independent Living." *Journal of Rehabilitation* 62, no. 3: 14–22.

Wiener, Joshua, L. H. Illston, and R. J Hanley. 1994. *Sharing the Burden: Strategies for Public and Private Long-term Care Insurance.* Washington, D.C.: Brookings Institution.

Wiener, J. M., C. M. Sullivan, and J. Skaggs. 1996. *Spending Down to Medicaid: New Data on the Role of Medicaid in Paying for Nursing Home Care.* Washington, D.C.: Brookings Institution.

Williams, Judith K. 1993. "Case Management: Opportunities for Service Providers." State of Wisconsin Community Options Program, *Home Health Care Services Quarterly* 14, no. 1: 5–40.

Index

activities of daily living (ADLs): assistive devices and, 79, 81; criteria for identifying, 23, 29; effects of ADL disability, 38; personal services and, 3; scale, 3

adult day care, 3. *See also* long-term care

AIDS: in CMA caseload, 28; as component of disability, 24; in risk population, 26

Alzheimer's disease, public expenditures for study of, 51

Americans with Disabilities Act, 44

assisted living, xi, 1, 124–26, 127–30; advantages of, 124, 133; availability of, 130; comparisons with other arrangements, 129; consumer choice issues and, 126; continuing care retirement community, 125; definitions of, 125–26; financing-based classification of, 126–27; as home care replacement, 124, 126; informal care prospects, 50; management of, 126; potential market for, 130–31, 136; Medicaid (HCFA) and, 134; number of residences in existence, 124; provision of, 134–35; "supportive housing," 125; trends in, 133, 136; utilization of, 132–33; varieties of, 127–28

assistive devices, x, 81, 88–89, 94–95; ADLs and, 79, 81; case managers and, 94; case strategies for use of, 84–85; consumers and, 84–85, 87; cost/cost effectiveness of, 85–86, 92, 94; demonstration programs, 91, 93, 94; future prospects for, 92–95, 177–78; household organization and, 88; and link to health care, 82–83;

market for, 82, 83; personal safety and, 79, 81–82, 89–92; product development and distribution, 82–83; resistance to, 87–88; as substitutes for formal care, 86; technology and, 79–80; third-party payment for, 83, 84, 86, 91; training required for use of, 87. *See also* personal response systems

Berkowitz and Gratton, on reliability of cost data, 24

Biagi, on families' provision of long-term care, 42

Brody, on families' provision of long-term care, 42

Brookings-ICF, on trends in health care expenditures, 149–50, 151

Burwell and Jackson, on patterns in consumer home-care financing, 150

Cantor, on age distribution among adult children acting as parents' caregivers, 36

Caro, on main themes of home and community-based care, 16

case management: cost of, in Massachusetts, 169; insurance companies' use of, 170–72; limits of role in consumer-directed models, 169–70; Medicare and, 172; as professional specialty, 173–74; public vs. private, 170; in publicly funded programs, 168

case management, private, 170–72; as element of long-term care coverage in California, 171

199

About the Authors

ROBERT MORRIS, D.S.W., is Kirstein Professor Emeritus, Brandeis University. He is currently co-editor of the *Journal of Aging and Social Policy* and a senior research fellow at the University of Massachusetts at Boston. He was editor-in-chief of the first comprehensive *Encyclopedia of Social Work and Welfare* and has written or edited numerous books and articles on social welfare and gerontology. With Francis Caro, he developed the concept of a social/health maintenance organization. He has been president of the Gerontological Society of America, consultant to numerous governmental and health or welfare agencies, and an officer of nonprofit social agencies. He is a fellow of the American Association for the Advancement of Science, the American Public Health Association, and the Gerontological Society of America.

FRANCIS G. CARO, PH.D., is professor and director of the Gerontology Institute at the University of Massachusetts at Boston. His current research emphases are productive aging, community-based long-term care, and evaluation research on interventions involving older people. He is the co-author of *Quality Impact of Home Care for the Elderly* and *Family Care of the Elderly*. He edited *Readings in Evaluation Research* and co-edited *Achieving a Productive Aging Society*. He is a co-editor of the *Journal of Aging and Social Policy*.

JOHN E. HANSAN, PH.D., is co-founder and coordinator of Odyssey Forum, an ad hoc group of social policy analysts, economists, social workers, and researchers interested in advancing humane social welfare policies. He also volunteers as the resource development director for the National Association of Retired and Senior Volunteer Programs. A gerontologist, he devoted fifty years to administering human service programs at the local, state, and national levels. He is the co-editor, with Robert Morris, of *The National Government and Social Welfare: What Should Be the Federal Role?*